Internet Guide
to Cosmetic Surgery
for Women

Internet Guide to Cosmetic Surgery for Women

M. Sandra Wood

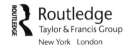

Routledge
Taylor & Francis Group
New York   London

First published by

The Haworth Information Press®, an imprint of The Haworth Press, Inc., 10 Alice Street, Binghamton, NY 13904-1580.

This edition published 2012 by Routledge

Routledge
Taylor & Francis Group
711 Third Avenue
New York, NY 10017

Routledge
Taylor & Francis Group
2 Park Square, Milton Park
Abingdon, Oxon OX14 4RN

PUBLISHER'S NOTE
This book has been published solely for educational purposes and is not intended to substitute for the medical advice of a treating physician. Medicine is an ever-changing science. As new research and clinical experience broaden our knowledge, changes in treatment may be required. While many potential treatment options are made herein, some or all of the options may not be applicable to a particular individual. Therefore, the author, editor, and publisher do not accept responsibility in the event of negative consequences incurred as a result of the information presented in this book. We do not claim that this information is necessarily accurate by the rigid scientific and regulatory standards applied for medical treatment. **No warranty, express or implied, is furnished with respect to the material contained in this book. The reader is urged to consult with his/her personal physician with respect to the treatment of any medical condition.**

PUBLISHER'S NOTE
Due to the ever-changing nature of the Internet, Web site names and addresses, though verified to the best of the publisher's ability, should not be accepted as accurate without independent verification.

Cover design by Jennifer M. Gaska.

Library of Congress Cataloging-in-Publication Data

Wood, M. Sandra.
   Internet guide to cosmetic surgery for women / M. Sandra Wood.
     p. cm.
   Includes bibliographical references and index.
   ISBN-13: 978-0-7890-1066-7 (hc. : alk. paper)
   ISBN-10: 0-7890-1066-6 (hc. : alk. paper)
   ISBN-13: 978-0-7890-1067-4 (pbk. : alk. paper)
   ISBN-10: 0-7890-1067-4 (pbk. : alk. paper)
   1. Surgery, Plastic—Computer network resources.   2. Women—Surgery—Computer network resources. 3. Internet addresses. 4. Web sites.
   [DNLM: 1. Surgery, Plastic. 2. Internet. 3. Reconstructive Surgical Procedures—methods. 4. Women.] I. Title.

RD119.W66 2005
025.06'617952—dc22

               2004031067

CONTENTS

Acknowledgment

The author would like to thank Lillian R. Brazin for her enthusiastic support and valuable comments and feedback concerning content and organization of this book.

ABOUT THE AUTHOR

M. Sandra Wood, MLA, MBA, AHIP, FMLA, is Librarian, Reference and Database Services, The George T. Harrell Library, The Milton S. Hershey Medical Center, The Pennsylvania State University College of Medicine, Hershey, Pennsylvania. She has over three decades of experience as a medical reference librarian, including the areas of general reference services, management of reference services, database and Internet searching, and user instruction. Ms. Wood has been widely published in the field of medical reference and is Editor of *Medical Reference Services Quarterly, Journal of Consumer Health on the Internet,* and *Journal of Electronic Resources in Medical Libraries* (Haworth). She is Editor or Co-Editor of several books, including *Women's Health on the Internet, Health Care Resources on the Internet: A Guide for Librarians and Health Care Consumers, Men's Health on the Internet,* and *Cancer Resources on the Internet.* She is a member of the Medical Library Association and the Special Libraries Association, and has served on the MLA's Board of Directors as Treasurer. Ms. Wood is also a Fellow of the Medical Library Association.

ABBREVIATIONS

AACD	American Academy of Cosmetic Dentistry
AACS	American Academy of Cosmetic Surgery
AAD	American Academy of Dermatology
AAFPRS	American Academy of Facial Plastic and Reconstructive Surgery
ABD	American Board of Dermatology
ABFPRS	American Board of Facial Plastic and Reconstructive Surgery
ABMS	American Board of Medical Specialists
ABO	American Board of Ophthalmology
ABOto	American Board of Otolaryngology
ABPS	American Board of Plastic Surgery
ABS	American Board of Surgery
ASAPS	American Society for Aesthetic Plastic Surgery
ASDS	American Society for Dermatologic Surgery
ASOPRS	American Society of Ophthalmic Plastic and Reconstructive Surgery
ASPS	American Society of Plastic Surgeons
FAQ	frequently asked question
FPSN	Facial Plastic Surgery Network
HON	Health on the Net
html	hypertext markup language
http	hypertext transfer protocol
NLM	National Library of Medicine
NOAH	New York Online Access to Health
PDF	portable document format
URL	uniform resource locator

SYMBOL KEY

🖈   Bulletin board

⊛   Chat room

🦷   Dentist locator

⬤   Discussion forum

✉   Message board

📷   Photo gallery

⚕   Physician locator

🤝   Support forum

⊕   Technician locator

Introduction

I am the original candidate for an "extreme makeover"—the TV show might have been named after me. Tummy tuck, belt lipectomy, liposuction, thigh lipoplasty, breast lift, spider veins, hair replacement, eyelid surgery (both undereye bags and drooping eyelids), wrinkle removal, facial liposuction for double chin—I would be a candidate for all of these procedures, and believe me, have considered all of them over the years and especially while researching and compiling this book. Ah, if I just had the money!

My interest in cosmetic surgery began many years ago. As someone who was constantly battling weight, I'd considered cosmetic surgery, but knew that it was not a solution to my problem. However, fifteen years ago, following the birth of my son, my stomach did not go back to where it had been. Not that it was ever truly "flat"—but after two cesarean sections, the stomach muscles were pretty much gone, and I started thinking about having a tummy tuck. I even got to the point of discussing it with a cosmetic surgeon about ten years ago, following an injury to my forehead which required thirty-one stitches. At a follow-up evaluation to determine whether scar revision would be necessary (it wasn't), I discussed both a tummy tuck and eyelid surgery with the cosmetic surgeon. To this day, I regret my decision not to have the surgery. I'm ten years older and have lost the time that I would have had feeling better about myself and also increased my surgical risk due to age. Also, time has done its damage—making additional procedures attractive.

I'm part of the baby-boomer generation and had children late in life; the latter has led to its embarrassing moments. I have been in a store where the clerk, talking to my son, referred to me as his grandmother. My son looked confused. However, it brought home the point to me that I'm not as young on the outside as I mentally feel on the inside. I want to think that being in my fifties is still young, and cosmetic surgery begins to sound more and more attractive.

It used to be that if you had cosmetic surgery, you didn't talk about it. It was something that just happened (e.g., you went away on a vacation and came back looking very "rested"). Basically, times have changed over the past ten years or so. Perhaps it's the fact that movie stars are talking openly about their cosmetic surgery. Or, possibly, it's because every week (sometimes every day), cosmetic surgery is the topic of a TV news or talk show. It's been the focus of several reality shows (*Extreme Makeover* and *The Swan*), and an FX show, *Nip/Tuck*. Or, it may be that the baby-boomer generation, looking to find its youth again—into the "antiaging" frame of mind—has brought cosmetic surgery into the mainstream. Everyday people, not just movie stars, are talking about cosmetic procedures, from the new "in" procedure, Botox, to the immensely popular surgical procedures of liposuction and breast enlargement.

So, if you (like me) are among the hundreds of thousands of women considering cosmetic surgery, how do you decide what procedure you want done? How do you find out information about the procedures and treatments that are available and how they are performed? How do you locate a qualified physician? These are the types of questions that this book is intended to help you answer.

The growth of the Internet during the 1990s has opened up ready access to all types of information. It didn't take long before the health care world realized that this was an appropriate way to transmit health care information to patients and consumers—including information about plastic/cosmetic surgery. The amount of information available on the Internet about cosmetic surgery and various over-the-counter cosmetic therapies is absolutely mind-boggling. Information is available online from professional associations, the government, educational institutions, physicians advertising their private practices, companies selling their products, physician locator services, and more. There is so much to sort through, that it becomes difficult and time-consuming to decide which sites to access, let alone which sites are reputable. This book is intended to help you locate quality information about cosmetic surgery on the Internet, guiding you to sites where you can begin your search.

The book is organized into eleven chapters. The first four chapters provide basic information. Chapter 1 introduces plastic and cosmetic surgery, including some definitions, cosmetic surgery as a "hot" trend, and statistics on the number of women in the United States having cosmetic surgery. Chapter 2 covers some Internet basics (if you are a beginner with the Internet, you may want to consider purchasing a separate Internet guide). This chapter helps you to evaluate sites, covers basic searching of the Internet, and recommends two megasites for consumer health information. Deciding to have cosmetic surgery involves both the decision of what procedure you want and choosing a physician. Chapter 3 covers selecting a physician, including board certification and membership organizations (and their Web sites). Much of the quality information available online comes from societies that credential physicians, so it seemed logical to include these sites in a discussion about board certification and credentialing. Chapter 4 introduces you to basic sites that provide cosmetic surgery information; it is divided into Web sites of professional organization sites (plus one university site) and commercial sites.

In the next four chapters, cosmetic procedures have been divided into "logical groupings"—body contouring; cosmetic surgery of the breast, cosmetic surgery of the face, head, and neck; and cosmetic surgery of the skin. Procedures are listed alphabetically under their "common" name, and there are cross-references from the technical names, plus plenty of suggestions to guide you to other related procedures. You will find many of the same sites listed in all chapters, just under different cosmetic procedures.

These chapters are followed by chapters on Web sites for hair transplantation for women and on cosmetic dentistry. The final chapter lists selected Web sites for professional organizations outside the United States. Cosmetic surgery has been popular outside the United States for many years, and women have traveled worldwide to clinics specializing in particular procedures. These organizations provide information that might prove useful should you be considering cosmetic surgery in another country.

One final caution. These sites are intended as starting points for you to gather information about cosmetic surgery and to locate the physician who might perform your cosmetic procedure. Ultimately, the decision of whether or not to have surgery should be made between you and your physician, and you are encouraged to discuss details of the procedure with him or her. You are urged to check your physician's credentials, including board certification and professional affiliations, and to evaluate previous work that he or she has done. Know the risks up front; make an informed decision.

Chapter 1

Cosmetic Plastic Surgery—The Basics

Thinking about having a cosmetic surgery procedure done? Not sure whether you want to let friends and relatives know you are considering having that nose reshaped, the bags under your eyes removed, or that tummy tuck to remove the bulge that's been there since your last child was born? Not sure about what is involved in the procedure, where to find information, or what doctor to perform the procedure? Afraid even to ask about cosmetic surgery because you don't know enough yet to ask intelligent questions?

Well, this book is for you. A wealth of information is available via the Internet, and, it can be accessed anonymously. As cosmetic surgery becomes more mainstream, the Internet is rapidly gaining popularity as the first resource to turn to for information. You can gather all sorts of background information about cosmetic surgery procedures, identify potential doctors to perform the procedures, and even chat online with others who have had cosmetic surgery, all from the comfort of your own home. The problem is, in fact, that there is too much information about cosmetic surgery on the Internet, and not all of it is accurate. This book is intended to guide you to quality sources of information about cosmetic surgery, but only you and a qualified physician can eventually make the decision as to whether or not you should undergo a cosmetic surgery procedure.

WHAT IS PLASTIC SURGERY?

Plastic surgery is the medical specialty involved with changing a person's appearance via surgery. Although people tend to think of plastic surgery in terms of its cosmetic use, in reality, according to the American Society of Plastic Surgeons, the majority of surgeries are reconstructive in nature. Cosmetic surgery is generally defined as surgery done for the purpose of improving appearance, i.e., it is plastic surgery for aesthetic purposes, while reconstructive surgery is done to correct or repair a defect, for example to correct a birth defect or repair an injury. The same procedure may be used either cosmetically or for reconstruction, and frequently the purpose of the surgery determines whether it is covered by health insurance. Most cosmetic procedures are not covered by insurance, although it's always good to check with your health insurance company.

Readers should keep in mind, however, that a procedure may be used either for cosmetic or reconstructive purposes, so this book will also be valuable for readers who need reconstructive surgery.

COSMETIC SURGERY IS A HOT TREND

Despite its cost, the days when cosmetic plastic surgery was limited to movie stars or the very rich and famous are long gone. Cosmetic surgery has boomed over the past decade or two, and several factors have contributed to this amazing increase in popularity. In recent years, people have become more open about having cosmetic surgery—it has become the "in" thing to do. Perhaps it's the aging baby-boomer set that doesn't want to admit it is aging; or, perhaps it's the increasing number of movie stars admitting—actually, being very open about the fact—that they have had cosmetic plastic surgery. The topic of cosmetic plastic surgery is much more out in the open than ever before. People that might not have considered cosmetic surgery several years ago are increasingly deciding to "go under the knife."

Cosmetic Surgery and Celebrities

The Internet is loaded with sites that discuss cosmetic surgery procedures of celebrities. Several sites list the stars, what procedure was done, and before and after pictures.[1,2] Included are, to name only a few, Pamela Anderson, Drew Barrymore, Cher, Heather Locklear, Madonna, Demi Moore, Anna Nicole Smith, Sharon Stone, and Raquel Welch. The search engine Yahoo! even has a "Celebrity Plastic Surgery" category among its directories.[3]

In fact, several sources go so far as to say that virtually everyone in Hollywood has had cosmetic surgery of some form or another. Although some are still reluctant to admit that they've had surgery, the fact is that in Tinseltown, looks are everything, and since age eventually takes its toll, cosmetic surgery, from laser peels through liposuction, ultimately wins out.[4]

In recent years, however, as more TV and movie stars have begun talking about their cosmetic procedures, "ordinary," everyday people are opening up about their experiences. Almost all of the daytime talk shows have explored the topic, it is constantly mentioned on syndicated TV shows such as *Entertainment Tonight (ET)* and *Extra,* and it's been discussed on many primetime news shows and on ABC's *Good Morning America.*[5] In spring 2003, ABC TV introduced *Extreme Makeover* into its nighttime lineup of shows after the success of a pilot program in late 2002. This show takes ordinary people and offers them a free cosmetic surgery makeover; application forms for people wanting to participate in this program can be found on <http://www.abcnews.com>. Other networks are also offering shows about cosmetic surgery, including FX's *Nip/Tuck,* a drama based on the life of a single, eligible plastic surgeon; FOX network's *The Swan,* where women undergo cosmetic surgery and then compete in a beauty contest; and MTV's *I Want a Famous Face,* where patients undergo cosmetic surgery to look like a celebrity. Although these TV shows have popularized cosmetic surgery, many of the professional medical associations are concerned that they are unrealistic and do not disclose enough about the risks of surgery. Programs such as *60 Minutes* and *20/20* have aired "exposés" about the risks of cosmetic surgery and the need to carefully select your surgeon.

Baby-Boomer Generation

As the generation of baby boomers has aged, health and physical fitness have become priorities. Women (and men) want to look and feel good about themselves. Cosmetic surgery is one way to keep a youthful appearance, whether it's used to erase those wrinkles and lines that appear with age, or to reshape one's body when exercise alone won't do the job.

Recent reports from the Centers for Disease Control indicate that obesity in America has become a major health concern. Interestingly, the increase in gastric bypass surgery (stomach stapling), a treatment for morbid obesity, has helped promote cosmetic surgical procedures. The major weight loss from stomach stapling can result in the need for cosmetic surgery to tighten up the body and remove excess skin.

More and more younger adults, even teens, are choosing to have plastic surgery as a means of correcting what they view as "defects." The prevailing attitude is, "if you don't like it, fix it." In the heavy-duty world of corporate America, appearance is everything. The confidence gained as a result of cosmetic surgery might make the difference between being hired or not, between getting that promotion or not.

WHAT ARE THE NUMBERS?

How many people have cosmetic surgery each year? What are the most frequent procedures, and do women have certain procedures more frequently than men? Is age a consideration in cosmetic surgery? How much does it cost? These are all questions that come to mind when one is considering cosmetic surgery. After all, it is comforting to know that others have had the same cosmetic procedure that you are considering. Having some realistic expectation of both costs and results will help you to make your decision.

Answers to all of these questions, and more, can be found on the Internet. Perhaps the best source of statistics on cosmetic surgery is available on the Web site of the American Society of Plastic Surgeons (ASPS) <http://www.plasticsurgery.org> (*note:* this is the form that will be used in this book for locations on the Internet; you will learn more about Internet addresses—URLs—in the next chapter). Statistics are available on this site by year (currently, 1992, 1996, and 1996 to 2003); by type of procedure; and by age, sex, and ethnicity. Also given are national average physician fees for cosmetic procedures (it's interesting to compare 1992 versus 2003 average fees). These numbers are for procedures reported by "ASPS member plastic surgeons certified by The American Board of Plastic Surgery."[6]

The ASPS site includes many quick facts about cosmetic and reconstructive surgical and nonsurgical procedures. Press releases on the ASPS site for 2003 indicate that over 8.7 million cosmetic surgery procedures were performed in 2003, up 32 percent from over 6.5 million procedures in 2002. The top five surgical procedures were nose reshaping, liposuction, breast enlargement, eyelid surgery, and facelifts.

Looking only at cosmetic surgery procedures for women, it's interesting to note that the top five female cosmetic procedures in 2003, according to the ASPS, were liposuction (287,930), breast enlargement (254,140), nose reshaping (226,780), eyelid surgery (200,324), and facelifts (115,908). Overall, women accounted for 1,469,265 cosmetic surgeries, or 82 percent of the total cosmetic surgical patients.

The largest jump in demand, according to the ASPS, was for minimally invasive plastic surgery, which jumped 41 percent in 2003 to over approximately 7 million procedures (from over 4.8 million in 2002). The biggest "winner" here was Botox, with nearly 2.9 million procedures. Distant second and third, for both men and women, was chemical peeling and microdermabrasion. Women accounted for 87 percent of the procedures.

Another site that has excellent statistics for cosmetic surgery is the American Society for Aesthetic Plastic Surgery (ASAPS) <http://www.surgery.org>. Their statistics also reflect procedures performed by members of the association. According to the ASAPS, the top five cosmetic surgeries for women in 2003 were liposuction (322,975), breast enlargement (280,301), eyelid surgery (216,829), breast reduction (147,173), and nose reshaping (119,047). Women accounted for 87 percent of more than 8.2 million procedures performed.

Many other sites on the Internet include statistics for cosmetic surgery, both in the United States and worldwide. However, the statistics available from the ASPS and ASAPS will be listed for each procedure (where available) because of the structured reporting procedures for each group of physicians. Note that these statistics are updated each year by the ASPS and ASAPS, usually in March for the previous year.

If you are considering cosmetic surgery, you are definitely encouraged to log onto the ASPS site <http://www.plasticsurgery.org> and the ASAPS site <http://www.surgery.org> and check out the numbers—who's having what procedure done. It's reassuring to know that many, many other people have had the procedure(s) that you are considering.

HOW MUCH DOES IT COST?

One other really interesting piece of information provided by both the ASPS and ASAPS is the cost for cosmetic procedures. What is listed at each of these sites is the U.S. national average surgeon/physician fee. You should note that anesthesia, facilities (operating room, outpatient surgicenter), and other expenses are not included, and that variables such as geographic location are not included. In 2002, over $7 billion were spent on physician fees for cosmetic surgery according to the ASPS. For 2003, the ASAPS reports over $9.3 billion spent.

WHY READ THIS BOOK?

Every woman wants to feel good about herself. It is a proven fact that a positive self-concept is linked to how you look and feel. How you look can be enhanced by cosmetic surgery. The decision to have cosmetic plastic surgery is a big step. It involves a physical change that will alter not only how you will look at yourself, but also how others will look at you. There are risks with surgery. In addition, the surgical costs are normally not covered by health insurance.

As you begin to evaluate whether or not you might want to undergo cosmetic surgery, you should gather as much information as possible so that you can make an informed decision. Although many people have had cosmetic surgery, you might not know anyone who can tell you of their experience; or, even if you know someone who has had a cosmetic procedure, you might not feel comfortable asking him or her about it. Locally, you will find that many plastic surgeons hold clinics to explain procedures. These informational meetings are usually a way of advertising and promoting procedures at their clinics. Even before attending such a meeting, knowing what is involved in a cosmetic procedure will help you to evaluate and ask good questions.

This is where the Internet comes in to play. Besides the information that your doctor will give to you, the Internet is perhaps your best source for information about cosmetic procedures. However, the Internet can be overwhelming in itself because of the quantity of information—there is so much available that it can be confusing, not all of it is accurate, and some can be actually misleading. This book will help you to identify Internet resources you can trust. The following chapters will cover basic Internet searching, finding a doctor, and how to locate information about specific cosmetic surgical and nonsurgical (minimally invasive) procedures. You'll learn about evaluating information from a Web site, selecting a "credentialed" physician, and locating information about specific procedures.

Ultimately, the choice of whether or not to have cosmetic surgery is yours, and yours alone. Input from family and friends and your doctor will all influence your decision, but the better informed you are about the surgical procedure, along with risks and complications, the better your decision will be. Resources in this book are intended to lead you to quality information to help you in your decision-making process. However, the information found in this book and on the Internet is not a substitute for the advice of your cosmetic surgeon, who is best qualified to evaluate you (your medical/physical condition) and determine whether you are a candidate for the cosmetic procedure you wish to have.

NOTES

1. Plastic People Page. Available: <http://www.geocities.com/hollywood/7990/plastic.html>. Accessed: August 20, 2004.

2. "Hollywood and Cosmetic Surgery." Available: <http://www.streamingsurgeries.com/hollywood/cosmetic_surgery_hollywood.html>. Accessed: August 23, 2004.

3. Yahoo! "Celebrity Plastic Surgery." Available: <http://www.yahoo.com/Society_and_Culture/People/Celebrities/Plastic.Surgery/>. Accessed: August 23, 2004.

4. "Looking Like a Celebrity. Plastic Surgery at the Front Lines of Glamour." ABCNews.com. Available: <http://printerfriendly.abcnews.com/printerfriendly/Print?fetchFromGLUE=trueandGLUESer...>. Accessed: May 28, 2003. (No longer available online.)

5. Pozniak, Alexa. "Face Off Over Face-Lifts. Experts Say 'Not So Fast' to Face-Lifts for 30-Somethings." ABCNews.com. Available: <http://printerfriendly.abcnews.com/printerfriendly/Print?fetchFromGLUE=trueandGLUESer...>. Accessed: May 28, 2003. (No longer available online.)

6. American Society of Plastic Surgeons. Available: <http://www.plasticsurgery.org>. Accessed: April 16, 2004.

Chapter 2

The Internet—Where to Begin

Finding information about cosmetic surgery on the Internet is easy; finding the right information on the Internet is a bit trickier. In fact, finding too much information on the Internet is, perhaps, the biggest problem. Literally millions of "hits" come up when doing a general search on "plastic surgery" via Internet Explorer or Netscape. Hundreds of thousands of sites can be located on individual procedures such as liposuction and Botox. The amount of information available is absolutely mind-boggling and extremely confusing. So confusing that you can be tempted to simply give up before you really start. The idea of having to wade through thousands of sites can be a real turnoff to continuing your search.

This is when knowing where to start searching and how to locate the best Web sites becomes valuable both in terms of time and quality of information. It's really important to be selective in what you look at on the Net. Using the simple tips listed in this chapter, along with going to the sites targeted later in this book, will give you the necessary know-how to find accurate information about procedures that you're interested in and help you to find a qualified physician located near you.

THE INTERNET

This book assumes a basic knowledge of the Internet—that you know it is a large, worldwide computer network (actually, it's a network of networks) that allows users to access information from around the world. Some basic information about Web addresses (hyperlinked sites on the Internet) will be given in this book. However, if you are a new Internet user ("newbie") and need more extensive information about the Net, you are advised to consult a basic Internet search guide such as *The Internet for Dummies*.[1] The second assumption is that you, the reader, have access to the Internet either at home, through a public library, from an "Internet café," or through some other location.

INTERNET ADDRESSES

The Internet and the World Wide Web (WWW, or simply "the Web") are not the same thing, although many people use these terms interchangeably. The Web uses a system of links between documents, or pages of information, that have been placed on a computer using hypertext markup language (html). The standard for linking to these documents is called hypertext transfer protocol (http), which is the prefix that you will see listed at the beginning of most Internet addresses. The locations for these documents, called "Web sites," are given addresses, known as URLs—for uniform resource locators. Throughout this book, you will see URLs listed in a standard format, consisting of the document format or protocol (http), followed by the host computer, directory, and file name, surrounded by angle brackets to set off the address. It will appear like this:

<protocol://host.domain.suffix/directory/file.extension>

For example, in the address <http://www.nlm.nih.gov/medlineplus/breast reconstruction.html>, the protocol is http, followed by ://www, which tells you this is a Web address; the domain is the National Library of Medicine at the National Institutes of Health, which is a government agency (.gov); the directory is MedlinePlus; the file name is breastreconstruction; and the file extension is html. All Web addresses will be listed this way, surrounded by angle brackets (< >). When you are searching for a Web address, everything gets typed in as the site information except the angle brackets.

As you begin searching the Internet, you need to remember that the Web is "fluid"—sites are constantly being updated, changed, added, and deleted, all of which leads to outdated sites and dead links. Dead links are the result of a change to a file name or site address. When you encounter a dead or broken link, you should delete information at the end of the address—e.g., the /directory or /filename.htm part of the address—and use only the host.domain.suffix part of the address. From there, you can search the site for the specific Web page or document that you are looking for. If you still cannot access the site, the whole site may have changed addresses, in which case you would need to do a Net search as described in Searching via Your Internet Browser in this chapter.

"GOOD" VERSUS "BAD" INFORMATION: EVALUATING WEB SITES

Whether you are an experienced computer user or someone just getting started with the Internet, some cautions are in order. A general subject search using any Internet browser will bring up hundreds of thousands of "hits"—sites that presumably include some information on cosmetic surgery. Unfortunately, the first sites that appear on the list may not be the "best" sites. In fact, the first sites that appear may have paid to have their site listed first. Sites that look relevant and appear attractive may actually contain incorrect or even dangerous information. Anyone can create a Web site that appears authoritative—from a former cosmetic surgery patient to your teenage daughter. As you scroll down the screen looking at the sites you've located, you may find that you've located totally inappropriate sites—some terminology in cosmetic surgery may actually lead you to pornography sites.

At minimum, quality, authoritative Web sites should be evaluated for the following:

- *Who created the site.* The person or group responsible for the content should be identified, along with a way to contact them. Credentials of the creator should be listed (e.g., education, experience, institutional affiliation).
- *Currency/last update.* The last update of the site should be listed; sites not frequently updated should be skipped. Are links to other sites still working?
- *Seal of approval.* Several national and international organizations have been created to accredit Web sites. One such organization is the Health on the Net Foundation (HON) at <http://www.hon.ch>. HON is an international Swiss organization that guides Internet searchers to reliable and useful medical and health information. The Utilization Review Accreditation Commission (URAC) <http://websiteaccreditation. urac.org> is an American organization that accredits quality health Web sites.
- *Bias.* Sites that give only one viewpoint (e.g., discuss a cosmetic procedure without listing risks) should be avoided. Does the site sell products or advertise a physician's clinic? Is it sponsored by a drug company?

- *Intended audience.* Web sites may be created for medical profession-als (physicians, nurses) or for consumers (e.g., patients, prospective patients, general public).
- *Look at the domain name.* The Web site address itself can be helpful in evaluating a site. The ending of the address indicates the location, e.g., "gov" is a U.S. government site, "org" is an organization, and "edu" is an educational institution (however, a tilde, or "~," in the "edu" address in-dicates personal Web space within the educational institution and could be a student's Web site).
- *Presentation/typos.* Does this Web site look like it was put together in haste—i.e., are there a lot of typographical errors? Is it easy to navi-gate; are pages linked logically? Overall, how well is it presented graphically?

Not all of these points must be present in a Web site for it to be considered a good or valuable site, but if in doubt, use these guidelines to determine how trustworthy it is.

Sites selected for inclusion in this book have been evaluated by the author based on the previous criteria. Not all of the sites selected meet all of the crite-ria. An attempt was made to select sites with quality content that would be representative of the types of sites found on the Internet, including organiza-tions, government, and commercial sites.

BASIC INTERNET SEARCHING

Each Internet searcher seems to have a favorite way to search the Internet. Some people just use the "Search" feature on their browser (e.g., Internet Explorer, Netscape), and input a search term (e.g., liposuction). Others have a favorite search engine, such as Ask Jeeves, Google, or Ya-hoo!. Still others have favorite megasites that they've bookmarked in spe-cial subject areas (e.g., MedlinePlus might be bookmarked for medicine and health care information). Although each of these methods might pro-vide some useful information, a combination is the best approach. Meth-ods described in this chapter are

- searching via your Internet browser,
- searching via a search engine directory, and
- searching via megasites.

Of these methods, searching megasites is preferable. However, since most people are more likely to be familiar with search engines or using their Internet browser, those will be briefly described first, followed by several recommended megasites to be used as starting points. Ultimately, though, you will be encouraged to use the recommended sites in later chapters of this book.

SEARCHING VIA YOUR INTERNET BROWSER

Internet browsers such as Netscape and Internet Explorer each have a "Search" feature that allows you to input a search term and get a list of "hits" on your topic. Subscribers to commercial services such as America Online (AOL) will also find a search feature on their home page. Although this appears to be the easiest method for finding information, it is the least recommended, and potentially, the most hazardous. For example, this author recently searched Netscape (which features Google) using "cosmetic surgery"—and found too many "hits" to look through. "Sponsored Links" appeared first (links that pay to be at the top), followed by "Matching Results"—in no particular order, although there were a high number of ".com" sites (commercial sites). Searching for "plastic surgery," "liposuction," and "Botox" brought up similarly lengthy lists. Clearly, the amount of information is overwhelming. How would you make a good choice on what links to follow, what sites to access? This is definitely *not* recommended as a good way to begin. So, in the hopes of persuading readers to take a different approach, what alternatives are available?

SEARCHING VIA A SEARCH ENGINE DIRECTORY

Many search engines are available on the Internet. A search engine can either be "man made" or a robot—a computer doing the search based on preprogramming. These search engines can be used in two ways. The first method is similar to a Web browser; however, this is not a recommended approach. A recent search of "cosmetic surgery" in Google, a popular search engine, resulted in 1,500,000 "hits"—so many sites that it was impossible to make a good selection of what site to visit. Some of the more popular search engines are listed in Table 2.1; use of these engines resulted in extensive lists of "hits" on cosmetic surgery topics, in no particular or-

TABLE 2.1. Selected search engines

Search Engine	URL
AlltheWeb	<http://www.alltheweb.com>
AltaVista	<http://www.altavista.com>
Ask Jeeves	<http://www.ask.com>
Google	<http://www.google.com>
HotBot	<http://www.hotbot.com>
LookSmart	<http://www.looksmart.com>
Mamma	<http://www.mamma.com>
Teoma	<http://www.teoma.com>
Yahoo!	<http://www.yahoo.com>

der other than sponsored sites being listed first. Again, while some good sites might be found this way, it is not the recommended approach. There are so many commercial and special interest sites to sort through that it's difficult to identify quality information.

A better approach is to use the directories that have been created within many of these search engines. These directories gather together information on general subject areas. Directory searching in Google, LookSmart, Lycos, Netscape Web Directory, and Yahoo! is described as follows (and, yes, some of these search engines are "oldies" but still "goodies").

Google
<http://www.google.com>

As mentioned, direct searching is available in Google, but it's recommended to go to Google's directory. Select "Google Directory," then "Health," then "Medicine," then "Surgery," and finally "Cosmetic and Plastic." As you can see, cosmetic surgery is really buried within the "Health" directory. However, once you've reached this level, access points include directories (listings of physicians), organizations, patient education (procedures), and surgeons and clinics. The surgeons and clinics section is organized by country, and within the United States, by state; links here go to physicians' individual Web sites.

LookSmart
<http://www.looksmart.com>

In LookSmart, you can begin by searching "cosmetic surgery" in the "Directory." A list of sites comes up, but if you scroll to the bottom, a list of "Related Directory Categories" shows both "Plastic and Cosmetic Surgery" and "Cosmetic Surgery and Plastic Surgery"—both going to the same page. Links are then available to specific cosmetic procedures.

Lycos
<http://www.lycos.com>

Lycos is one of the older search engines on the Internet, and although overshadowed recently by Google, it is still a good search engine. A general search on Lycos initially might seem like a good approach, but "cosmetic surgery" brings up over 1 million records, with no apparent logic as to what's listed first. This is where the Lycos Web Directory comes in handy. Select "Web Directory," then "Health," then "Medicine," then "Surgery," and finally "Cosmetic & Plastic." This brings up a page of links that go to sponsored listings (note: commercial sites); Categories, including surgeons and clinics (note: commercial sites), directories, organizations, etc.; and Web sites (note: commercial sites intermingled with organizations, etc.). Within this grouping, the most useful is "Organizations," which has links to professional organizations including non-U.S. groups. "Directories" and "Surgeons and Clinics" can both be used as physician locators.

Netscape—Web Directory
<http://www.netscape.com>

To access Netscape's Web Directory, first click on "Search," which brings up the page with the Web Directory. From there, select "Health," then "Medicine, then "Surgery," and then "Cosmetic and Plastic." Subcategories include organizations, patient education, publications, and reconstructive surgery. Netscape is also a sponsor of an open access initiative called the dmoz Open Directory Project <http://www.dmoz.org>, which has access categories similar to Netscape's Web Directory.

Yahoo!
<http://www.yahoo.com>

In Yahoo! scroll to the Web Site Directory, and from there choose "Health," then "Procedures and Therapies," then "Surgeries," and then "Cosmetic & Plastic." Specific links are available for "Breast Augmentation," "Breast Reduction," and "Liposuction." Just for fun, you can also locate information on celebrities having plastic surgery from the Web Site Directory on Yahoo's home page by selecting "Society and Culture," then "People," then "Celebrities," and finally "Plastic Surgery."

SEARCHING VIA A MEGASITE

The recommended way to begin searching on the Internet for information about cosmetic surgery procedures is to begin with a megasite. A megasite is defined here as a site that contains large amounts of information or links to information on other Web sites. These sites do not create the information, but provide organized access to information on other Web sites. The sites listed as follows were selected from a group of excellent resources; it's just not possible to include an exhaustive list. The resources and links included in these sites will get you started in the right direction—gathering quality information to help you make a decision about whether or not to have a cosmetic surgical procedure.

Ask NOAH About: Plastic and Cosmetic Surgery
<http://www.noah-health.org>

NOAH (New York Online Access to Health) is a megasite created by a cooperative of libraries in New York City. Originally intended as a guide to health care information for residents of New York City, this resource has grown into a major site recognized worldwide as providing quality health information. From the main NOAH page, select "Health Topics" and then "Plastic and Cosmetic Surgery," or go directly to <http://www.noah-health. ong/en/procedures/surgery/cosmetic/>. On this page (see Figure 2.1) are links to information about specific procedures; definitions; complications, including insurance and safety issues; care and treatment; and information resources. Most links go to consumer sites provided by professional organizations and university health centers; all resources have been evaluated by librarians before being linked into the NOAH page. This is a great place

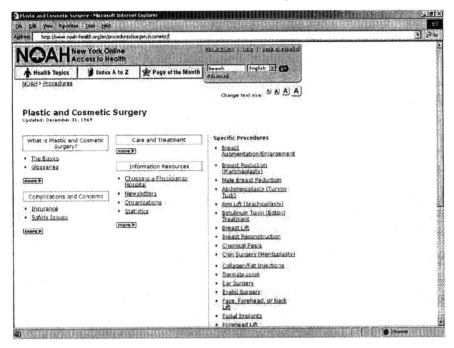

FIGURE 2.1. NOAH Page on Plastic and Cosmetic Surgery
<http://www.noah-health.org/en/procedures/surgery/cosmetic/>
Reprinted with permission of New York Online Access to Health.

to start your search for quality information, and it also contains links to resources for choosing a physician or a hospital. A Spanish version of NOAH is available.

MedlinePlus
<http://medlineplus.gov>

MedlinePlus is made available by the National Library of Medicine (NLM), the world's largest medical library. It is "designed to help you find appropriate, authoritative health information" at both the consumer and professional level. The site contains health news, drug information, an illustrated medical encyclopedia, a dictionary, links to medical databases such as MEDLINE, and links to other Web sites containing health information on over 600 diseases. NLM clearly posts its selection guidelines for these materials, including quality of content, noncommercial sources, and availability/maintenance of the Web pages. This site is considered to be the premier Web site for consumer health materials, and thus is an excellent starting place for locating information on cosmetic and plastic surgery.

Once in MedlinePlus, select "Health Topics" and then the letter "P." On the "P" page, select "Plastic & Cosmetic Surgery." This page brings together the majority of links in MedlinePlus about cosmetic surgery (see Figure 2.2). From the latest news and general information through links to specific procedures, treatment, and statistics, this page is a great place to start gathering information about the cosmetic procedures that interest you. A majority of the links on this page go to pages produced for consumers by professional organizations, including the American Society of Plastic Surgeons and the American Academy of Facial Plastic and Reconstructive Surgery (more on these later in this book). From this page, you can also link to other relevant MedlinePlus pages on topics such as

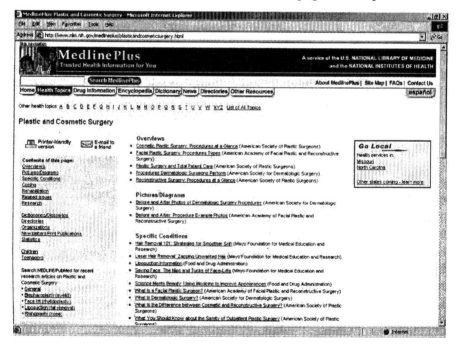

FIGURE 2.2. MedlinePlus Page on Plastic and Cosmetic Surgery
<http://www.nlm.nih.gov/medlineplus/plasticandcosmeticsurgery.html>

Botox, breast implants, scars, and varicose veins. A Spanish version of MedlinePlus is available, also.

MOVING ON TO SPECIFIC SITES

As you begin to become familiar with the primary sites that are linked to these megasites, you will then begin to recognize them as authoritative and go directly to those sites. For example, you will find that sites such as the American Society of Plastic Surgeons and the American Society for Aesthetic Plastic Surgery will be prominently featured within these megasites, along with other professional organizations, government sites, and some commercial sites. You will then be ready to begin looking for information on specific procedures at the specific sites listed in later chapters of this book.

NOTE

1. Levine, John; Young, Margaret Levine; and Baroudi, Carol. *The Internet for Dummies,* 9th Edition. Hoboken, NJ: Wiley Publishing, 2003 (or later edition).

Chapter 3

Selecting a Cosmetic Surgeon

As you begin to think about cosmetic plastic surgery, you will need to learn about procedures that are available and to make a decision on who will perform your cosmetic surgery. If you are anxious to begin learning about the procedures, then skip ahead to later chapters in this book, where you will find Internet sites about many popular cosmetic surgery procedures. However, many of the recommended sites are, in fact, produced for prospective patients (consumers such as yourself) by the professional membership associations of cosmetic surgeons, so it's important that you understand the role these organizations play in certifying that your prospective surgeon has the proper training and experience to perform cosmetic procedures. This chapter will help you to select a cosmetic surgeon by leading you to information about both the selection process and physician credentials. So, while you may actually decide first on what cosmetic procedure you want, understanding the qualifications and medical/surgical specialties that are involved with cosmetic surgery may actually influence the procedure that you ultimately select.

HOW TO FIND A GOOD COSMETIC SURGEON

If you've been thinking about having cosmetic surgery performed, you may already have a physician in mind. For example, you might have looked in your local phone book, checked the yellow pages, and made a selection based on what's listed in the doctor's ad. In fact, you may have already checked out several prospective surgeons on the Internet because many doctor's offices are listing their Web address (URL) in their phone book or newspaper ads, and you've gone online to their Web site. It's become fairly routine now for doctors to place Web site information in the local yellow pages just so potential patients (like you) can check information online in the privacy of their own homes.

Or, you may have a friend or have met someone who has had plastic surgery, and asked them whether or not they would recommend the physician who performed their surgery. Person-to-person referral is still one of the best ways to locate potential surgeons, as you can get firsthand information about how well your friend liked his or her experience, from comments about the doctor to whether he or she had any problems or difficulties following the surgery. You also have an opportunity to see how the surgery actually turned out. After all, cosmetic surgery is a very personal decision, and you will need to feel comfortable with both the surgeon and the results of the surgery.

The recent development of the Internet has greatly expanded the ability to locate and select a cosmetic surgeon, both locally and at a distance. Although most people will select a local surgeon to perform their cosmetic procedure, you can now use the Internet to find an expert worldwide, should you decide that you want to travel to another location for your surgery.

Some basic guidelines to consider in selecting a cosmetic surgeon:

- Check your surgeon's credentials. Board certification, medical licensure, and membership in professional organizations are all relevant to how well your surgeon is qualified.
- What surgery center/hospital does your surgeon use? Is it accredited?
- Check your surgeon's malpractice history.
- How many years has your surgeon been practicing? How many procedures has he or she done of the type you are considering?
- Ask to see examples (photos) of the work that he or she has done.
- Do you feel comfortable with this surgeon? How well does he or she listen to what you say you want done? Does he or she answer all of your questions?

These are some of the factors to consider in selecting the cosmetic surgeon that is right for you. The Internet has many sites that actually provide checklists and questions for you to ask your prospective surgeon. A few are briefly listed as follows, with more detailed descriptions of these and other Web sites in later chapters of this book.

American Academy of Cosmetic Surgery—Choosing
a Cosmetic Surgeon
<http://www.cosmeticsurgery.org/Patient_Center/choosing_a_
cosmetic_surgeon.html>

American Society of Plastic Surgeons—Make the Right Choice
<http://www.plasticsurgery.org/find_a_plastic_surgeon/Making-
an-Informed-Decision.cfm>

Facial Plastic Surgery Network—How to Find and Choose
a Great Surgeon
<http://www.facialplasticsurgery.net/findingasurgeon.htm>

CREDENTIALS/BOARD CERTIFICATION

Much of the decision process depends on personal opinion and a certain "comfort level." Perhaps more important, though, is the need to evaluate the credentials of the doctor who will perform your cosmetic procedure. Cosmetic surgery requires special training and certification by appropriate professional boards before a physician is considered to be fully qualified. A physician who performs cosmetic surgery procedures should list "board certified" as one of his or her credentials. It's important to look for a board certified doctor; having a medical degree (MD or DO) is not enough. However, you should also know which professional board has certified the physician, i.e., what is the physician's medical specialty? Would you want a radiologist to perform a liposuction procedure? Or, would you feel comfortable with your family physician performing breast enlargement? The radiologist and family physician will be board certified in their own specialty, but that does not qualify them to perform cosmetic plastic surgery. Thus, a physician indicating that he or she is "board certified" is insufficient information for you to make a decision. What board has certified them?

In recent years, as cosmetic plastic surgery has become more popular, physicians who are board certified in "other" specialties have taken quick courses on cosmetic surgery and begun to perform cosmetic procedures. They don't need to deal with insurance companies for reimbursement (after all, you are paying for the procedures and they can charge what they want), and this has become a way to increase/augment their income. Although these physicians may do a fine job, you should be fully aware of a physician's qualifications and track record before undergoing any surgical procedure.

ABMS Board Certification

Board certification implies a basic knowledge and skill level, frequently determined by a number of years of postgraduate medical training and experience (residency), passing an examination, and maintaining skills through continuing education. When searching for a qualified physician, evaluating credentials such as board certification is essential. However, there is not just one board that certifies physicians who perform cosmetic procedures, and this can be very confusing as you evaluate credentials.

The American Board of Medical Specialists (ABMS) is an organization made up of twenty-four approved medical specialty boards that grant certification to physicians (MDs and DOs) who have completed an approved training program (residency) and passed an examination. Similar boards approve specialty training in other countries. Although you will find board certified physicians from many specialties offering cosmetic procedures, you should look for a physician certified by one of the following specialty boards: American Board of Plastic Surgery, American Board of Dermatology, American Board of Ophthalmology, American Board of Otolaryngology, and American Board of Surgery. Physicians from other specialties may also perform specialized types of cosmetic surgery. Also, other boards exist for subspecialties (e.g., facial cosmetic surgery), but they represent further specialization and do not replace an ABMS board certification. The American Board of Plastic Surgery is listed first, with the other specialties then listed alphabetically.

American Board of Plastic Surgery
<http://www.abplsurg.org/>

The mission of the ABPS is to "promote safe, ethical, efficacious plastic surgery to the public by maintaining high standards for the examination and certification of plastic surgeons as specialists and subspecialists." Information about the board certification process and examination information is available. This site is primarily for physicians specializing in plastic surgery, but is of interest to health care consumers because standards are listed. The Board is a member organization of the American Board of

Medical Specialists and is the primary certifying body in the United States for plastic surgeons.

The Plastic Surgeon Referral Service is the place to start your search for a surgeon. From the main page <http://www.plasticsurgery.org>, choose "Find a Plastic Surgeon" and connect to the membership directory of the American Society of Plastic Surgeons (ASPS)—a society in which you would expect your cosmetic surgeon to be a member. Or, go directly to <http://www.plasticsurgery.org/findsurg/finding.htm>. All surgeons listed here are board certified by the American Board of Plastic Surgery and/or the Royal College of Physicians and Surgeons of Canada. Besides surgeons in the United States and Canada, members are listed from sixteen countries from around the world.

The initial "Find a Plastic Surgeon" page allows you to search by last name, state, Canadian province, and country. If you choose a state from the pull-down menu, you can then search by city and/or procedure. Surgeons' names are linked to more complete information: name and address, phone, fax, gender, board certification, insurance/financing options, and procedures that the surgeon offers. If you have a particular surgeon that you wish to check out, or you are looking for a surgeon in a particular state or city, this is the first directory to search.

American Board of Dermatology
<http://www.abderm.org>

The American Board of Dermatology is accredited by the ABMS to certify physicians as specialists in dermatology; dermatologists must complete postgraduate training and pass an examination to become board certified. Dermatologists evaluate and treat patients with "disorders of the skin, hair, nails and adjacent mucous membranes." According to this site, "Dermatologists also manage cosmetic disorders of the skin, including hair loss, scars, and the skin changes associated with aging." Thus, many dermatologists will perform cosmetic procedures involving the skin and face.

If you select "Verifying Certification," you are linked to a page that gives directions for mailing $25 to the ABD for written verification. For free verification, follow the link at the bottom to the ABMS Web listings, or call the number listed for verbal verification. If you are looking for a physician to perform a cosmetic skin procedure, in addition to being certified in dermatology, you will want to look for credentials like membership in an organization such as the American Society for Dermatologic Surgery and the American Academy of Dermatology.

American Board of Ophthalmology
<http://www.abop.org>

The American Board of Ophthalmology is one of twenty-four specialty boards recognized by the ABMS. It certifies ophthalmologists in the United States. The ABO page refers you to the ABMS page <http://www.abms.org> for online verification of certified ophthalmologists (free, but you must register), and provides directions for obtaining written verification (for a fee). In addition to being certified by the ABO, you would also want your physician to be a member of the American Society of Ophthalmic Plastic and Reconstructive Surgery, which requires further specialization.

American Board of Otolaryngology
<http://www.aboto.org>

The American Board of Otolaryngology (ABOto) is the organization recognized by the ABMS to certify otolaryngologists, the specialty that deals with head and neck surgery. Cosmetic and reconstructive plastic surgery of the head and neck may be performed by an otolaryngologist. From this site, you can click on "Diplomates" and then "Verification" to get free online verification; written verification is available for a $25 fee. You would also want your surgeon to be a member of an organization such as the American Board of Facial Plastic and Reconstructive Surgery, which requires further specialization.

American Board of Surgery
<http://www.absurgery.org>

"The ABS is an independent, non-profit organization with worldwide recognition. It is one of the twenty-four certifying boards that are members of the American Board of Medical Specialties." To check on board certification for your physician, you are directed to link to the ABMS Web site, or to make your inquiry via mail or phone to the ABS. Since this board certifies general surgeons, you would want your surgeon to have further specialization and training in cosmetic surgery.

Subspecialty Board

American Board of Facial Plastic and Reconstructive Surgery
<http://www.abfprs.org/>

Some plastic surgeons limit their practice primarily to cosmetic, plastic, or reconstructive surgery of the face. The American Board of Facial Plastic and Reconstructive Surgery (ABFPRS), established in 1986, is "dedicated to improving the quality of facial plastic surgery available to the public by measuring the qualifications of candidate surgeons against certain rigorous standards." To achieve certification by the ABFPRS, the surgeon must have completed an accredited residency program with training in facial plastic surgery, and be certified by the American Board of Plastic Surgery and/or the American Board of Otolaryngology, or in Canada, the Royal College of Physicians and Surgeons of Canada in otolaryngology or plastic surgery. In addition, he or she must pass a special examination and also present "100 surgical cases in facial plastic and reconstructive surgery for each of the previous two years."

Part of this Web site is aimed at physicians interested in becoming certified by the ABFPRS. However, if you select "Who's Board Certified" at the top of the page, you can access the list of certified facial plastic surgeons. Simply click to accept the Disclaimer (absolves the board of liability), and a map of the United States and Canada comes up. After selecting your state, access is then available by physician name or city. For a surgeon's address and phone number, you must click on the electronic directory of members of the American Academy of Facial Plastic and Reconstructive Surgery (AAFPRS). After a notice that you are moving to the AAFPRS Web site, you can search for a physician by state (lists all in the state), zip code, country, or last name of physician. You should be aware that this directory also contains surgeons who are members of AAFPRS but not certified by ABFPRS.

Professional Membership Organizations

There are many professional membership organizations that cosmetic plastic surgeons elect or qualify to join. Membership in such organizations carries with it both prestige and an implied level of competence. Many membership organizations, such as the American Society of Plastic Surgeons, require that members be board certified and have taken additional continuing education courses to be a member. You will want your surgeon to be both board certified and a member of a professional organization related to cosmetic surgery.

These membership organizations' Web sites are featured throughout this book because they provide information to prospective patients about cosmetic surgery procedures and offer free doctor-locator services. The Web sites also give advice on how to evaluate and select a cosmetic surgeon, so these sites are featured as physician selection sites (as follows). A more comprehensive description of these Web sites will appear in Chapter 4.

LOCATING/SELECTING A COSMETIC SURGEON ONLINE

The Web abounds with sites that claim to be able to locate cosmetic surgeons throughout the United States and worldwide. As you look through the Internet, and in fact with some commercial sites listed in this book, there are many sites that claim to have a "physician locator." Use of commercial sites to locate your cosmetic surgeon is *not* recommended. In fact, if you decide to explore these sites, you will often find only one or two physicians listed per state—making these lists useless. Rather, you should limit your search for a qualified cosmetic surgeon to listings in professional membership organizations. In general, Web sites of professional organizations have the best, most comprehensive, and up-to-date physician locator lists—as you would expect, since cosmetic surgeons want to be able to list membership in these organizations as one of their credentials. Table 3.1 is a selected list of U.S. cosmetic surgery associations that offer physician-locator information. Although they are U.S. based, some of them have Canadian and/or worldwide membership. Each of these sites will be described later in Chapter 4, "Basic/Core Sites on Costmetic Surgery for Women." A selected list of organizations from other countries is given in Chapter 11 for non-U.S. readers, or for U.S. readers who are contemplating surgery outside the United States.

NEXT: BASIC COSMETIC SURGERY SITES ON THE INTERNET

So, you've made a preliminary decision about the surgeon you might wish to perform your cosmetic surgery procedure. However, you want to know more about the procedure that you *think* you want and what alterna-

TABLE 3.1. Professional organization Web sites with physician locators

Organization/URL	From Home Page Select:
American Academy of Cosmetic Surgery <http://www.cosmeticsurgery.org>	Patient Center, then Find a Surgeon Near You
American Academy of Dermatology <http://www.aad.org>	Find a Dermatologist
American Academy of Facial Plastic and Reconstructive Surgery <http://www.aafprs.org>	Patients>Physician Finder
American Society for Aesthetic Plastic Surgery <http://www.surgery.org>	Find a Surgeon
American Society for Dermatologic Surgery <http://www.asds-net.org>	Find a Dermatologic Surgeon
American Society of Ophthalmic Plastic and Reconstructive Surgeons <http://www.asoprs.org>	Membership Directory
American Society of Plastic Surgeons <http://www.plasticsurgery.org>	Find a Plastic Surgeon

tives might be available. When you go for a preliminary meeting with your surgeon, you want to know enough to ask the right questions and to understand his or her answers. In short, you want to be knowledgeable and informed. Chapter 4 will get you started on the Internet by reviewing basic sites about cosmetic surgery.

Chapter 4

Basic/Core Sites
on Cosmetic Surgery for Women

This chapter focuses on basic, core Web sites that provide information on women's cosmetic surgery procedures. Out of the hundreds of thousands of sites available, relatively few could be selected for this book. Selection was primarily based on criteria listed in Chapter 2 for evaluating information on the Internet, including reputation of the source, currency, nonbiased information, and presentation. Many of the sites selected for inclusion in this chapter are produced by U.S. professional associations (.org); however, it was impossible to ignore the highly commercial nature of cosmetic surgery, which is reflected in the large number of commercial sites on the Internet. Some of these commercial sites are quite well done and provide extensive, unique, and relevant information. Therefore, selected representative commercial sites are included where it was felt that they would help you make an informed decision about your cosmetic surgery. It should be noted, though, that while the Web sites of professional organizations might be preferred over commercial sites, one of the roles of these organizations is to serve as an advocate for their members, and thus their Web sites are used to publicize cosmetic surgery and to guide you to the offices of their cosmetic surgeon members.

It makes sense to check out some of these sites initially to familiarize yourself with the procedures and terminology before seeking further information from an individual physician's site, or even before contacting a local cosmetic surgeon. The more information you find before selecting a physician, the better, as you will be able to evaluate what a physician posts on his or her Web site and you will be better able to ask questions of the physician when you meet and talk with him or her about your potential surgery.

This chapter is organized into two primary sections. First is a group of sites that I consider "feature sites," which provide general information. These are primarily the sites of the membership organizations of physicians who perform cosmetic surgery, including the American Society of Plastic Surgeons; one originates from a medical school. These sites are top-rated locations that feature a variety of procedures. They offer basic information about many cosmetic procedures; a few focus on one area of the body (e.g., the eye).

The second section consists of commercial sites that offer basic information about a variety of cosmetic procedures. Commercial sites make up the majority of the hundreds of thousands of sites about cosmetic surgery you will find on the Internet. Although many of the commercial sites on the Internet are the sites of individual doctors or groups of doctors, a few sites provide general cosmetic surgery information. Several are listed as examples.

In addition to the sites listed in this chapter, you are encouraged to begin your search with the appropriate sections in the two megasites that were listed in Chapter 2: NOAH and MedlinePlus.

Ask NOAH About: Plastic and Cosmetic Surgery
<http://www.noah-health.org/en/procedures/surgery/cosmetic/>

MedlinePlus—Plastic and Cosmetic Surgery
<http://www.nlm.nih.gov/medlineplus/plasticandcosmeticsurgery.html>

GENERAL SITES (.ORG) ON COSMETIC SURGERY PROCEDURES FOR WOMEN

American Academy of Cosmetic Surgery
<http://www.cosmeticsurgery.org>

The American Academy of Cosmetic Surgery (AACS) represents surgeons in many medical and surgical disciplines, all involved with cosmetic surgery. This site contains information for member surgeons, patients, and a media center (see Figure 4.1). Select "Patient Center" to get to the page where you can choose "Learn About a Cosmetic Procedure," get information about "Choosing a Cosmetic Surgeon," or "Find a Cosmetic Surgeon Near You." At the time of evaluation, the site included patient information for twelve procedures. The physician locator seemed a bit limited (e.g., primarily major cities in the United States were represented); it can be searched by last name, city, and/or state.

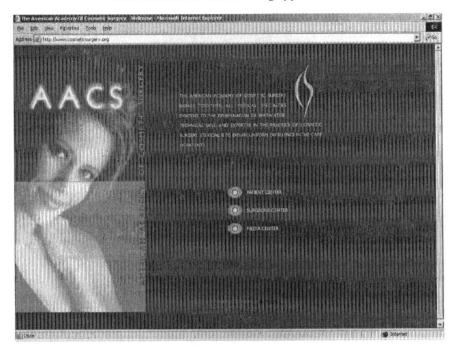

FIGURE 4.1. American Academy of Cosmetic Surgery Home Page
<http://www.costmeticsurgery.org>
Reprinted with permission of American Academy of Cosmetic Surgery.

American Academy of Dermatology
<http://www.aad.org>

The American Academy of Dermatology (AAD) is "dedicated to achieving the highest quality of dermatologic care for everyone." The AAD, with a membership of over 13,700, "is the largest, most influential and most representative of all dermatologic associations." Its Web site has information for both members and patients.

To access patient information about cosmetic surgery, select "Public Resource Center" from the home page, and then, on the lower left-hand side of the page, select "Publications" and then "Pamphlets." Pamphlets cover everything from dermatologic conditions to cosmetic surgery. Additional useful information for patients can be found in "Press Releases" (select under "News & Events," on left side of page).

Selecting "Find a Dermatologist" from the top bar of any page links you to "Find a Dermatologist Search" with access to a membership of 13,000 dermatologists in the United States and Canada. This is searchable by state, area code, zip, last name, city, or country.

American Academy of Facial Plastic and Reconstructive Surgery
<http://www.aafprs.org>

The American Academy of Facial Plastic and Reconstructive Surgery (AAFPRS) is a specialty society of the American Medical Association representing over 2,700 members worldwide. AAFPRS members are board certified surgeons who deal with facial, head, and neck surgery.

The AAFPRS Web site states, "Trust Your Face to a Facial Plastic Surgeon." From the main page (see Figure 4.2), in the "Patients" section, select "Procedures." From that page you can then select the "Virtual Exam Room" that allows you to highlight the part of the face that you want surgery on, and then you can get information on the procedure. Or, "Procedure Types" links you directly to information on cosmetic surgical procedures of the face that are online adaptations of the academy's patient brochures. On the left-hand side, "Before and After" shows a photo gallery of selected procedures; in the FAQs, you will find a glossary that defines medical terms, plus some statistics are available.

The AAFPRS's "Physician Finder" can be selected from the home page or from the "Patients" page. It is a membership directory of U.S. and Canadian facial plastic surgeons, and can be searched by state, and then zip code and radius in miles from the zip; there are also some international members.

American Society for Aesthetic Plastic Surgery
<http://www.surgery.org>

The American Society for Aesthetic Plastic Surgery (ASAPS) says that it is "the leading organization of plastic surgeons certified by the American Board of Plastic Surgery who specialize in cosmetic surgery of the face and body." Founded in 1967, it has 1,900 members in the United States and Canada, as well as members in other countries. The ASAPS's site (see Fig-

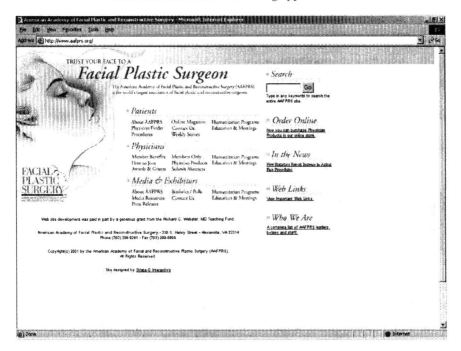

FIGURE 4.2. American Academy of Facial Plastic and Reconstructive Surgery Home
   Page
<http://www.aafprs.org>
Reprinted with permission of American Academy of Facial Plastic and Reconstructive
   Surgery.

ure 4.3) is a public information site providing cosmetic plastic surgery information; a section of the site is reserved for ASAPS members. Five major sections of the site guide potential patients to quality information.

Selecting "Medical Professionals" from the main page guides you to information about the society, including its mission and qualifications for
membership in ASAPS, and a link to statistics. Selecting "Procedures"
from the main page leads you to a page of over twenty procedures, from
which you can select the procedure(s) that interests you. Procedures include: botulinum toxin injections, breast augmentation, breast lift, breast
reduction, chemical peel, eyelid surgery, facelift, facial implants, fat injection, forehead lift, hair transplantation, lipoplasty, microdermabrasion,

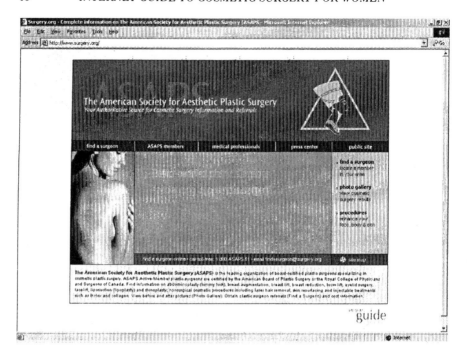

FIGURE 4.3. American Society for Aesthetic Plastic Surgery Home Page
<http://www.surgery.org>
Reprinted with permission of American Society for Aesthetic Plastic Surgery.

nose reshaping, skin resurfacing, and tummy tuck. Several of the topics are available in Spanish. Some procedures, such as lipoplasty, have more detailed information, including who should have the procedure, information on the technique, risks, "Your Surgical Experience" (before and after surgery information), links to pictures ("Photo Gallery"), and "Find a Surgeon." Other procedures, such as hair transplantation, have only brief information on the procedure, benefits, and other considerations. "Photo Gallery" can also be selected from the home page.

The "Find a Surgeon" is one of the better doctor locators. You can locate a surgeon by name and/or city/state; by distances up to fifty miles from your zip code; or in locations outside the United States. The list of members is extensive.

This site has excellent information about cosmetic surgical procedures and is one of the two main sites that make statistics available. Statistics can be accessed from the main page by selecting "Media" and then "Statistics" (available for every year from 1997 through 2003, at the time of this review). This is certainly a location that you should check out for both background information and selecting a physician.

American Society for Dermatologic Surgery
<http://www.asds.net>

The American Society for Dermatologic Surgery was founded "to promote excellence in the subspecialty of dermatologic surgery and to foster the highest standards of patient care." This is a membership organization of board certified dermatologists. The ASDS site (see Figure 4.4) has both a "members only" section and information for prospective patients. If you "mouse over" "Patients," you can then choose links to "Skin Care Corner," "Dermatologic Surgical Procedures," "Fact Sheets," "Before and After Photos," and more.

The "Dermatologic Surgical Procedures" section contains fact sheets on over twenty-five specific procedures. This site features everything from treatments for aging skin, spider veins, and warts to hair restoration. Although you may think of this site for "skin-only" surgery, you should know that liposuction, a body contouring procedure, was developed by dermatologic surgeons, and the ASDS site contains extensive information about this procedure.

"Find a Dermatologic Surgeon" can be selected from the main page or from "Procedures." It is searchable by state or country and by procedure.

American Society of Ophthalmic Plastic
and Reconstructive Surgery
<http://www.asoprs.org>

The American Society of Ophthalmic Plastic and Reconstructive Surgery (ASOPRS) is a membership organization of ophthalmologists who are certified by the American Board of Ophthalmology and have additional training and experience in plastic surgery of the "eyes and their sur-

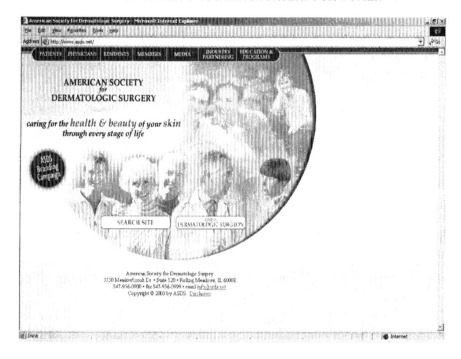

FIGURE 4.4. American Society for Dermatologic Surgery Home Page
<http://www.asds.net>
Reprinted with permission of American Society for Dermatologic Surgery.

rounding structures," and have passed a specialized examination. There are "over 400 national and international members" of the society.

The ASOPRS Web site includes basic information about cosmetic surgery of the eyelids; this is accessed via a "Patient Information" link at the bottom of the page. A "Membership Directory" can be selected at the bottom of the page or via a link on the left-hand side. This directory is searchable by state, and a small number of countries.

American Society of Plastic Surgeons
<http://www.plasticsurgery.org>

The American Society of Plastic Surgeons (ASPS) was founded in 1931. It is the "largest plastic surgery specialty organization in the world."

Members of ASPS are board certified by either the American Board of Plastic Surgery or the Royal College of Physicians and Surgeons of Canada. "The mission of ASPS is to advance quality care to plastic surgery patients by encouraging high standards of training, ethics, physician practice and research in plastic surgery." The importance of board certification is discussed in Chapter 3.

The ASPS Web site (see Figure 4.5) provides public education about cosmetic and reconstructive plastic surgery, along with information specific to members of ASPS (password protected for members). The most prominent links on the page are "Find a Plastic Surgeon," "Learn About Procedures," and "News Room," but you should check out all of the links. The site is crammed with everything from statistics about the number of procedures performed by ASPS members to information about qualifications required of board-certified surgeons and how to select a physician.

The home page for "Learn About Procedures" is a document called "Procedures at a Glance," which gives general information about most cosmetic surgery procedures. This, and the other pages, are called "brochures" because they are converted for online viewing from ASPS brochures. This overview of procedures includes a brief definition of each procedure (including the popular name of the procedure, e.g., abdominoplasty is a tummy tuck); length of time to perform the procedure; anesthesia used; whether it's an inpatient or outpatient procedure; risks involved; and recovery time. Procedures listed include abdominoplasty, breast enlargement, breast lift, chemical peel, eyelid surgery, facelift, hair replacement, liposuction, nose surgery, and more. From this page, you can link to more detailed information about nearly twenty procedures.

Selecting "Find a Plastic Surgeon" links you to the "Plastic Surgeon Referral Service." "All of the surgeons listed through the service are ASPS members who are board-certified by the American Board of Plastic Surgery and/or the Royal College of Physicians and Surgeons of Canada." This directory is searchable by a doctor's last name, procedure, address, city and state, or distance from a zip code. This plastic surgeon locator is the most comprehensive listing available on the Internet and recommended as the first place to begin locating a qualified surgeon in your area.

From the "News Room" on the main page, you can link to pages about cosmetic and reconstructive surgical procedures, official ASPS news releases, and more. A photo gallery is also available. This site has a site search feature and extensive links, making it easy to navigate within the site.

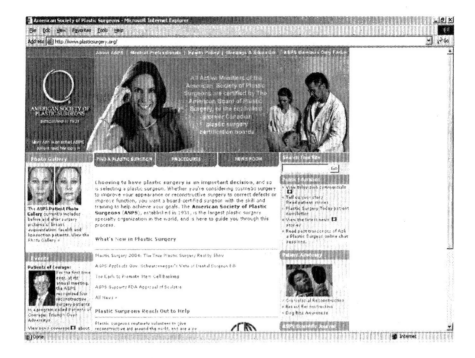

FIGURE 4.5. American Society of Plastic Surgeons Home Page
<http://www.plasticsurgery.org>
© 2004 American Society of Plastic Surgeons. All rights reserved. Learn more at
    <www.plasticsurgery.org>.

Virtual Hospital—A Patient's Guide to Plastic Surgery Procedures
<http://www.vh.org/adult/patient/surgery/plasticsurgery/index.html>

The Virtual Hospital is a "digital library of health information," developed and maintained by faculty and staff at the University of Iowa Medical Center. It provides information at both the patient and professional level, presented in the form of electronic books. The general page on plastic surgery links to FAQs, an alphabetic list of glossary terms, plus more complete descriptions of selected procedures. Information has been internally reviewed by Iowa faculty and is neutral in presentation.

GENERAL SITES (.COM) ON COSMETIC SURGERY PROCEDURES FOR WOMEN

Cosmetic Surgery FYI
<http://www.cosmeticsurgeryfyi.com>

Cosmetic Surgery FYI, developed by Einstein Medical, Inc., is primarily a cosmetic surgeon locator site; however, it contains extensive information about numerous cosmetic surgery procedures, including: breast augmentation, liposuction, abdominoplasty, rhinoplasty, hair transplantation, facelifts, and Botox injections. The list of cosmetic surgeons on this site is not extensive, but information about a wide variety of cosmetic procedures makes it a valuable resource. This is the "parent" site of a group of FYI sites about specific types of cosmetic surgery, several of which will be listed in later chapters by the surgical procedure.

Facial Plastic Surgery Network
<http://www.facialplasticsurgery.net>

"The Facial Plastic Surgery Network is dedicated to helping you obtain solutions to your facial aesthetic concerns." This site is produced by Enhancement Media, a company that has a group of "sister" sites on many cosmetic surgery topics. The site is easy to navigate, with links at the top of the home page to "Facial Procedures," "Choosing a Surgeon," "Procedure FAQ," "Anesthesia Information," a photo gallery, financing information, chat groups and discussion forums, and more (see Figure 4.6). The key page is "Facial Procedures," which has links to an extensive list of procedures, divided by type of procedure (e.g., skin). Information is similar to the site Yes They're Fake! which is also produced by the same company, just without the candid commentary. The information about each procedure is extensive, covering everything from the procedure itself to risks and complications. Especially useful is a link to a page about how to evaluate your physician's credentials. This site, and the other sites by Enhancement Media, are all interlinked and share chat groups and discussion forums. Chat groups and discussion forums are useful for online discussions about cosmetic procedures with other women who have had, or are contemplating, the same procedure.

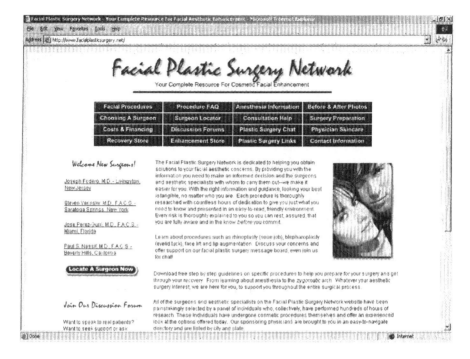

FIGURE 4.6. Facial Plastic Surgery Network Home Page
<http://www.facialplasticsurgery.net>
Reprinted with permission of Enhancement Media.

iEnhance
<http://www.ienhance.com>

iEnhance indicates that its "mission is to help people attain a more attractive body and image." The iEnhance site (see Figure 4.7) serves primarily as a locator service of "qualified plastic surgeons, cosmetic surgeons, dermatologists, cosmetic dentists and vision correction specialists." The site indicates that all physicians listed are board certified by the American Board of Plastic Surgery. The list of surgeons can be accessed by specialty, state or country, or doctor's last name. The site includes information on specific procedures (select "Procedures" at the bottom of the page; then select "Plastic Surgery" to bring up an extensive list). From the home page, you can select "Plastic Surgery," "Facial Plastic Surgery," "Dermatology," "Cosmetic Dentistry," or "Vision," where you will find featured articles and links to surgical procedures and more. The site also includes a photo gallery, message board, and financing information for patients.

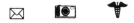

Medem
<http://www.medem.com>

The Medem Network, designed to facilitate physician-patient communication, maintains a "full range of patient education information from . . . partner societies and other trusted sources." The site includes information for physicians, patients, and industries (e.g., health plans and systems). Select "For Patients" from the home page, then "Browse Topics." Under "Therapies and Health Strategies," select "Plastic Surgery/Cosmetic and Reconstructive Procedures." Links from this page go to Insurance Issues, Plastic Surgery Basics, Procedures of the Breast, Liposuction, Other Cos-

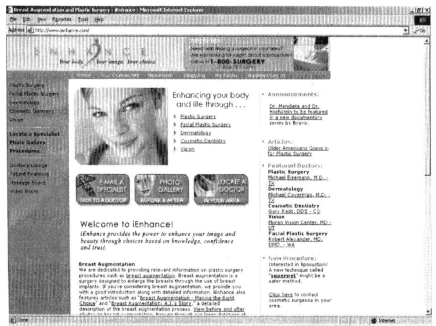

FIGURE 4.7. iEnhance Home Page
<http://www.ienhance.com>
Reprinted with permission of iEnhance.com.

metic Procedures, Statistics, etc. The majority of the material available from Medem was produced by organizations such as the American Society of Plastic Surgeons and the American Academy of Facial Plastic and Reconstructive Surgery.

Yes They're Fake!
<http://www.yestheyrefake.net>

This is the "fun" site that was mentioned at the beginning of this chapter. Yes They're Fake! is a refreshingly candid and irreverent site (see Figure 4.8), created by a woman who has undergone multiple cosmetic procedures. The actual content (surgical procedure, risks, complications, anesthesia, etc.) duplicates what can be found on the Facial Plastic Surgery Network <http://www.facialplasticsurgery.net>. However, it's the personal

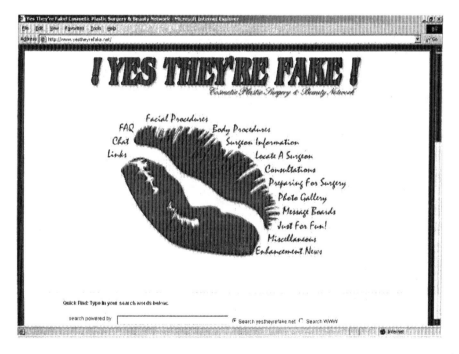

FIGURE 4.8. Yes They're Fake! Home Page
<http://www.yestheyrefake.net>
Reprinted with permission of Enhancement Media.

commentary that makes this site so unique and interesting. This site has "attitude."

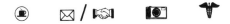

NEXT: INTERNET SITES FOR SPECIFIC COSMETIC SURGERY PROCEDURES

The Web sites in this chapter will be listed many times in the remaining chapters of this book, but you will be guided to specific cosmetic procedures within each Web site. One of your choices is to use these sites "in general"—to go directly to whichever site you have chosen (e.g., American Society of Plastic Surgeons or the American Academy of Facial Plastic and Reconstructive Surgery), and simply explore the many procedures and information located on each site. Or, you can go directly to the specific cosmetic surgery procedure in which you are interested by using the direct links in the remainder of this book. By dividing chapters into logical groupings by body site, you should easily find the procedure(s) that you are interested in; this will also allow you to browse for related procedures. Cross-references guide you within chapters, and the Index can also be used to locate the cosmetic procedure that you are considering.

Chapter 5

Body Contouring

This chapter covers body contouring procedures, or reshaping of the body. These procedures make up a large portion of the cosmetic surgery procedures performed on women. Although liposuction (lipoplasty) is the primary surgical procedure in this group, it also includes tummy tucks (abdominoplasty), buttock augmentation, and calf implants. Please follow cross-references, which lead to other sections in this chapter or to other chapters. In general, the "common" name rather than the technical name is used for a procedure.

Breast surgery—breast implants/augmentation, breast lifts, and breast reduction—is also considered body contouring. Because breast surgery is done almost exclusively in women and is so highly requested, it has been given a chapter of its own (see Chapter 6, "Cosmetic Surgery of the Breast").

BODY CONTOURING—GENERAL

Bermant Plastic and Cosmetic Surgery
<http://www.plasticsurgery4u.com>

This site is provided by Dr. Michael Bermant, a board certified physician in plastic surgery, who practices near Richmond, Virginia. Although the site is not well organized, it contains a wealth of information. Scroll until you get to "Body Sculpture" and then link to information on liposuction, thighplasty, tummy tuck, and more. The site subscribes to the HONcode principles.

Yes They're Fake!—Body Enhancement
<http://www.yestheyrefake.net/body_plastic_surgery.html>

This is a refreshingly candid site, created by a patient who has undergone cosmetic surgery herself. Go directly to the URL, or go to the main page <http://www.yestheyrefake.net>, and select "Body Procedures." The "Body Enhancement" page (see Figure 5.1) is an alphabetic list of approximately thirty cosmetic procedures, including procedures of the breast. Many of the procedures on this summary page are also listed individually later in this chapter and in Chapter 6.

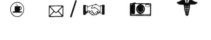

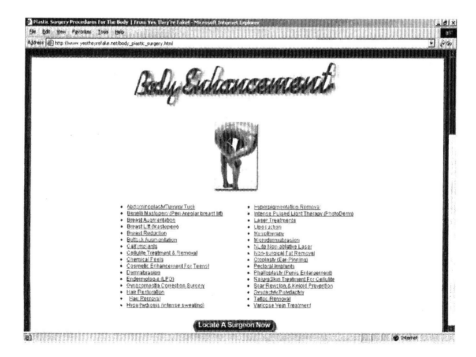

FIGURE 5.1. Yes They're Fake!—Body Enhancement
<http://www.yestheyrefake.net/body_plastic_surgery.html>
Reprinted with permission of Enhancement Media.

ABDOMINAL LIPOSCULPTURE (LIPOSUCTION)

Abdominal liposuction removes fat from the abdomen and reshapes the abdominal area. *See also* LIPOSUCTION; TUMMY TUCK (ABDOMINOPLASTY).

iEnhance—Abdominal Liposculpture
<http://www.ienhance.com/procedure/default.asp>

Go directly to the "Procedures" page and select "Plastic Surgery," then under "Abdomen" select "Abdominal Liposculpture (Liposuction)." Includes basic information such as patient selection, surgical procedure, risks, and postsurgical recovery.

ARM LIFT (BRACHIOPLASTY)/ ARM LIPOSUCTION

Brachioplasty, also called upper arm lift, is the surgical reduction of the upper arm to remove loose, hanging skin that may occur due to aging or weight loss. With arm liposuction, fat is first suctioned out of the arm; follow-up surgery may be required to remove excess skin.

2003 statistics:
ASAPS:	10,595	(10,361 in women)
ASPS:	8,890	(6,805 women)

eMedicine—Liposuction, Upper Arms
<http://www.emedicine.com/plastic/topic31.htm>

This is an article by Dr. JoAnne Lopes that describes liposuction in the upper arms. Although it's a bit technical, it describes the procedure and methods of assessing patients as candidates for upper arm liposuction.

iEnhance—Arm Liposuction
<http://www.ienhance.com/procedure/default.asp>

From the "List of Procedures," select "Plastic Surgery" and then, under "Arms," select "Arm Liposuction" and/or "Arm Lifts/Brachioplasty." Gives basic information about the procedure, risks, what to expect post-surgery, questions to ask your surgeon, and costs.

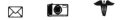

BELT LIPECTOMY

Belt lipectomy is described as doing a facelift on the entire torso. It is an extensive procedure and not offered at many locations (both sites selected here originate with the University of Iowa).

2003 statistics:
ASAPS: 10,964 lower-body lifts   (9,107 in women)

University of Iowa Plastic Surgery—Belt Lipectomy—Lower Body Lift—Central Body Lift
<http://www.surgery.uiowa.edu/surgery/plastic/beltlipectomypage. html>

This page describes belt lipectomy as a "face-lift for the trunk" and lists several names for the procedure (e.g., body lift, circumferential lipectomy). Five groups of patients are described as good candidates for this procedure. Each group is discussed, and there are extensive before-and-after pictures. Reasons are also given for patients who would not be good candidates for this surgery. The process at the University of Iowa is described, including the surgery, postoperative care, results, and complications. Information for out-of-town patients is given.

Virtual Hospital—Belt Lipectomy
<http://www.vh.org/adult/patient/surgery/plasticsurgery/ beltlipectomy.html>

Belt lipectomy, which involves removal of excess skin and fatty tissue that surrounds the trunk or body, is described. Information is given on who would (or would not) make a good candidate for this procedure, which is complex and not offered in many places. Among the names for this procedure are body lift and torsoplasty.

BODY LIFT

See BELT LIPECTOMY.

BUTTOCK AUGMENTATION/IMPLANT

Buttock augmentation is a surgical procedure for reshaping and increasing the size of the buttocks, either to create a balanced look, or to simply enlarge the butt area. This is accomplished with either an implant (silicone) or through micro fat grafting. This procedure has become more in demand in recent years due to people wanting to look like celebrities, e.g., Jennifer Lopez.

2003 statistics:
ASAPS: 3,885   (2,804 in women)

Yes They're Fake!—Buttock Augmentation
<http://www.yestheyrefake.net/buttock_augmentation.htm>

This refreshingly candid site was created by a patient who has undergone cosmetic surgery herself. Go directly to the URL, or go to the main page <http://www.yestheyrefake.net>, select "Body Procedures," and then "Buttock Augmentation." The page describes the surgery and types of augmentation (implants versus micro fat grafting), recovery (including pre-op and post-op instructions), risks and complications, questions to ask, and more.

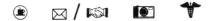

BUTTOCK LIPOSCULPTURE/LIPOSUCTION

Buttock liposuction removes fat from the buttocks and reshapes the buttock area.

2003 statistics:
ASAPS: 3,565   (3,450 in women)
ASPS: 2,411   (2,160 in women)

iEnhance—Buttock Liposculpture/Liposuction
<http://www.ienhance.com/procedure/default.asp>

From the "List of Procedures" select "Plastic Surgery" and then, under "Buttocks/Groin," select "Buttock Liposculpture/Liposuction." The page gives basic information about the procedure, risks, what to expect post-surgery, questions to ask your surgeon, and costs.

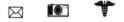

CALF IMPLANTS

Calf implants reshape the lower legs. In the procedure, an implant (such as silicone) is inserted into the leg to give it more shape and definition.

2003 statistics:
ASAPS: 1,170   (331 were women)

iEnhance—Calf Implants
<http://www.ienhance.com/procedure/default.asp>

From the "List of Procedures" select "Plastic Surgery" and then, under "Legs," select "Calf Implant." This page gives basic information about the procedure, risks, what to expect postsurgery, questions to ask your surgeon, and costs.

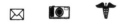

Yes They're Fake!—Calf Augmentation
<http://www.yestheyrefake.net/calf_augmentation_implants.htm>

This refreshingly candid site was created by a patient who has undergone cosmetic surgery herself. Go directly to the URL, or go to the main page <http://www. yestheyrefake.net>, select "Body Procedures," and then "Calf Implants." The page (see Figure 5.2) describes the surgery and types of augmentation (implants versus micro fat grafting), recovery (including pre-op and post-op instructions), risks and complications, questions to ask, and more.

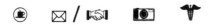

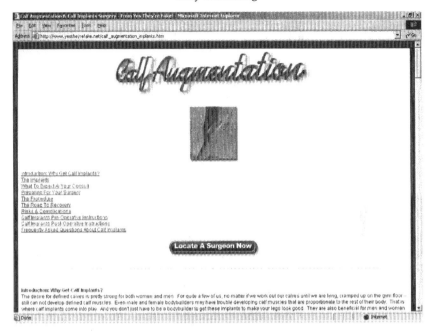

FIGURE 5.2. Yes They're Fake!—Calf Augmentation
<http://www.yestheyrefake.net/calf_augmentation_implants.htm>
Reprinted with permission of Enhancement Media.

LIPOSUCTION

According to the American Society for Aesthetic Plastic Surgery and the American Society of Plastic Surgeons, liposuction was the number one elective cosmetic procedure for women in the United States in 2003. Liposuction is defined by the ASPS as "a procedure that can help sculpt the body by removing unwanted fat from specific areas, including the abdomen, hips, buttocks, thighs, upper arms, chin, cheeks and neck."[1] By removing fat, weight loss occurs, but liposuction should not be considered solely as a weight-loss method. The best candidates for liposuction are women who exercise and eat the right foods, but may have stubborn areas of fat that just will not come off despite proper diet and exercise. Several methods of liposuction can be used, but the most common is tumescent liposuction, in which fluid containing lidocaine (an anesthetic) is injected into the area where fat is to be removed. This provides some local anesthesia and makes it easier for the cannula (a small tube used in this procedure) to break up fat and remove it.

Liposuction information is easily found on the Internet; in fact, a recent Google search brought up over 927,000 "hits." Sites that come up first on a general search are not always the best sites. Following are some recommended sites that include both professional and reviewed sites, along with a representative selection of commercial sites.

2003 statistics:

ASAPS:	384,626	(322,975 in women)
ASPS:	320,022	(287,930 in women)

American Academy of Cosmetic Surgery—Liposuction
<http://www.cosmeticsurgery.org/procedures/liposuction.asp? mn=pc>

Go directly to the page on liposuction (see Figure 5.3), or go to the main page <http://www.cosmeticsurgery.org> and select "Patient Center," then "Learning About a Cosmetic Procedure," then "Liposuction." Information includes who is a good candidate for surgery, risks, the surgical procedure, and postsurgery.

American Academy of Dermatology—Tumescent Liposuction
<http://www.aad.org/public/Publications/pamphlets/Liposuction. htm>

This AAD online pamphlet describes liposuction, focusing specifically on tumescent liposuction. The pamphlet describes the procedure and its benefits, indications for the surgery, and why a patient would choose a dermatologic surgeon for this procedure. Postsurgery and safety information are included.

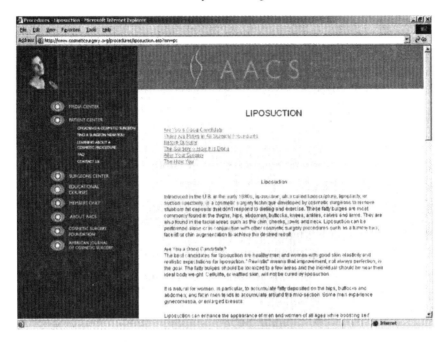

FIGURE 5.3. American Academy of Cosmetic Surgery—Liposuction
<http://www.cosmeticsurgery.org/procedures/liposuction.asp?mn=pc>
Reprinted with permission of American Academy of Costmetic Surgery.

American Society for Aesthetic Plastic Surgery—Liposuction (Lipoplasty)
<http://www.surgery.org/public/procedures-lipoplasty.php>

Go directly to this page (see Figure 5.4), or from the ASAPS home page, select "Public Site," then "Procedures," and "Liposuction." This page is set up such that you need to select "next" to get to all of the liposuction information on the site. This is an excellent place to begin; it contains everything from a description of various liposuction procedures to before-and-after surgery and potential complications. Contains illustrations, plus a photo gallery, and an extensive "Find a Surgeon" feature. This page is also available in Spanish.

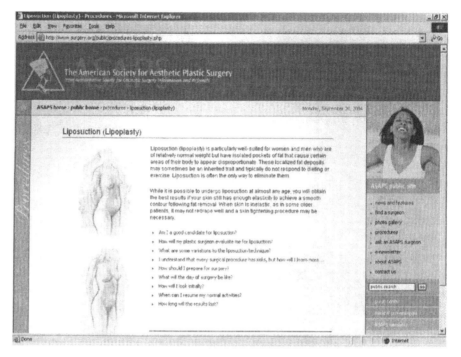

FIGURE 5.4. American Society for Aesthetic Plastic Surgery—Liposuction (Lipoplasty)
<http://www.surgery.org/public/procedures-lipoplasty.php>
Reprinted with permission of American Society for Aesthetic Plastic Surgery.

American Society for Dermatologic Surgery
<http://www.asds.net/skin_care_corner.html>
<http://www.asds.net/FactSheets/lipo_surgery.html>

The ASDS features liposuction information in several sections of its
Web page. "The Skinny on Liposuction" and the fact sheet on "Liposuction Surgery" contain unique but overlapping information promoting liposuction. The site claims that approximately one-third of all liposuction
procedures in the United States are performed by dermatologic surgeons.

American Society of Plastic Surgeons—Lipoplasty (Liposuction) <http://www.plasticsurgery.org/public_education/procedures/ Lipoplasty.cfm>

The ASPS public information page on liposuction (see Figure 5.5) includes surgery description, anesthesia information, technique variations, risks, postsurgical recovery, and before/after illustrations. This is one of the more extensive pages about liposuction and a top choice for beginning your search for information. This page is available in Spanish (choose Spanish from "Procedures" page or go directly to <http://www. plasticsurgery.org/public_education/procedures/Liposuccion.cfm>). You should also check out the description of the *tumescent technique* at <http://www. plasticsurgery.org/public_education/procedures/LiposuctionTumescentTechnique. cfm>.

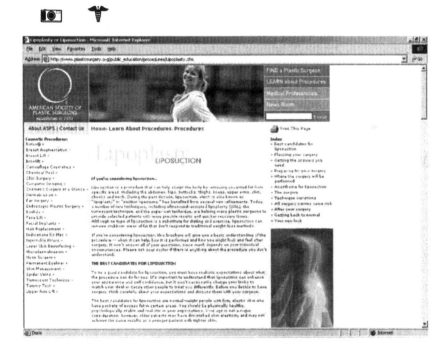

FIGURE 5.5. American Society of Plastic Surgeons—Lipoplasty (Liposuction) <http://www.plasticsurgery.org/public_education/procedures/Lipoplasty.cfm>

iEnhance.com
<http://www.ienhance.com>

This site separates its information about liposuction into specific areas of the body. Look elsewhere in this chapter under "Abdominal Liposculpture (Liposuction)"; "Arm Liposuction"; and "Buttock Liposculpture/Liposuction"; and in Chapter 7, "Cosmetic Surgery of the Face, Head, and Neck," under "Neck Lift/Neck Liposuction."

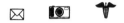

Lipoinfo.com
<http://www.lipoinfo.com>

This site is offered by Dr. Paul Weber of Ft. Lauderdale, Florida. It claims to be "the most comprehensive liposuction information site on the Internet," and very well may be. Information includes everything from the history of liposuction, definitions, and anatomy to details on the types of liposuction, procedures, anaesthesia, side effects, and before-and-after pictures. Dr. Weber has an extensive curriculum vitae that includes board certification in dermatology, specialized fellowship in dermatologic surgery, patented medical instruments, and a long list of publications. The site provides information for potential patients who evidently travel to Florida from throughout the United States and the world to have liposuction performed by Dr. Weber, so the site definitely has a commercial intent. However, Dr. Weber's presentation about liposuction, its proper use, and complications offers a unique perspective that is worth reading. The style is unique and offers information not available on other sites. Information in Spanish is available here, also.

LipoSite
<http://www.liposite.com>

LipoSite is an interactive chat site, offering you the opportunity to talk in real time to other people considering this procedure. The site also features message boards, statements of personal experiences, a photo gallery, and a physician locator (with a small number of participating surgeons). The extensive list of LipoSite Rules lists CompuMedical, L.L.C. (of Florida) as the site owner.

Liposuction 4 You
<http://www.liposuction4you.com>

This site is produced by Enhancement Media, a company that has a group of "sister" sites on many cosmetic surgery topics. The site is easy to navigate, with links that go to pages on "Your Anatomy," "Learn About Liposuction," "Surgery Information," "Road to Recovery," selecting a surgeon, costs and financing, links to professional organizations worldwide, and more. Within each page are links to fairly extensive information; for example, the surgical procedure page contains topics such as: "How much fat can be safely removed in one procedure?" and "Does fat 'grow back'?" Within "Plastic Surgeon Information" are links to help you research your surgeon and how to select a good surgeon. "Just for Fun" includes a chat room.

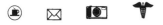

Liposuction Consumer Guide
<http://www.liposuction-consumer-guide.com>

The site includes basic information on liposuction, for example, types of procedures, benefits, risks, and questions to ask your surgeon. The site features a locator service to find a liposuction surgeon in your local area, but the list is not extensive.

LiposuctionFYI.com
<http://www.liposuctionfyi.com/index.html>

This is a special section of CosmeticSurgeryFYI.com that provides extensive information about the liposuction surgical procedure, whether you are a candidate for the procedure, risks, options available, and FAQs. It contains links to before/after photos. The commercial aspect is evident with a link to the Liposuction DocShop on each page, plus financing information.

MayoClinic.com—Liposuction: Considerations About Body Sculpting
<http://www.mayoclinic.com>

Go to the general Mayo Clinic site <http://www.mayoclinic.com> and do a site search for "liposuction." This page gives an honest appraisal of what liposuction can and cannot do, questions to ask your surgeon, techniques of liposuction (tumescent and ultrasonic), postsurgery information, and risks of the procedure.

Medem: Medical Library—Liposuction
<http://www.medem.com>

To get to the liposuction page, select "For Patients—Medical Library," then select "Plastic Surgery/Cosmetic and Reconstructive Procedures," and finally "Liposuction." The liposuction page links to six documents, all from the American Society of Plastic Surgeons. Some of the pages are no longer on ASPS's own Web site.

U.S. Food and Drug Administration, Center for Devices and Radiological Health—Liposuction Information
<http://www.fda.gov/cdrh/liposuction>

The Food and Drug Administration (FDA) regulates drugs (e.g., anesthetics) and medical devices, including equipment used to perform liposuction. The FDA site (see Figure 5.6) has basic information about liposuction and who performs the procedure, risks and complications, and "What can I expect" before, during, and after the surgery. Alternatives to liposuction are given. Information about where to report a problem can be found here. Anyone considering liposuction should go to this site to read about the risks/complications. Click "Printable Version of All Liposuction Information" or go directly to <http://www.fda.gov/cdrh/liposuction/complete.html> to get a printable version of all liposuction pages linked to this FDA page.

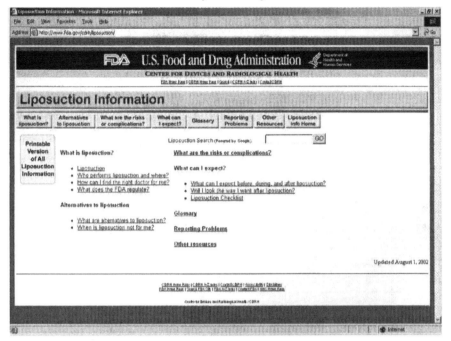

FIGURE 5.6. U.S. FDA—Liposuction Information
<http://www.fda.gov/cdrh/liposuction>

Yes They're Fake!—Liposuction
<http://www.yestheyrefake.net/liposuction.htm>

This refreshingly candid site was created by a patient who has undergone cosmetic surgery herself. Access the URL directly, or go to the main page <http://www.yestheyrefake.net>, select "Body Procedures," and then "Liposuction." The page describes the surgery, indications and contraindications for liposuction, risks and complications, and more. You are referred to a "sister" site—Liposuction 4 You <http://www.liposuction4you.com> (see separate listing).

THIGH LIPOSUCTION (THIGHPLASTY)/
THIGH LIFT

Thigh liposuction is the removal of fat to reshape the thigh; it can be done to remove fat deposits on both the inner and outer thigh area.

2003 statistics:

ASAPS:	8,806 thigh lifts	(8,563 in women)
ASPS:	5,615 thigh lifts	(5,322 in women)

iEnhance—Thigh Liposculpture
<http://www.ienhance.com/procedure/default.asp>

Link directly to the "Procedures" page and select "Plastic Surgery," then under "Legs" select "Thigh Liposculpture." This page includes basic information about thighplasty, from selection of patients and the surgical procedure through risks, postsurgery, and costs. A link to "Leg Lift" is incomplete and has photos only.

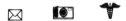

TUMMY TUCK (ABDOMINOPLASTY)

Tummy tuck (abdominoplasty) is a surgical procedure that removes fat and skin from the tummy area, while also tightening the abdominal muscles. Tummy tucks are often performed in conjunction with liposuction. Women should wait to have a tummy tuck until after their final pregnancy.

2003 statistics:

ASAPS:	117,693	(112,713 in women)
ASPS:	101,228	(95,644 in women)

American Academy of Cosmetic Surgery—Abdominoplasty
(Tummy Tuck)
<http://www.cosmeticsurgery.org/procedures/abdominoplasty_
tummy_tuck_.asp?mn=pc>

Go directly to the page on abdominoplasty, or go to the main page <http://www.cosmeticsurgery.org> and select "Patient Center," then "Learning About a Cosmetic Procedure," then "Abdominoplasty." Information includes who is a good candidate for surgery, risks, the surgical procedure, and postsurgery.

American Society for Aesthetic Plastic Surgery—Tummy Tuck <http://www.surgery.org/public/procedures-tummytuck.php>

The ASAPS page on tummy tucks (see Figure 5.7) has basic information about who is a good candidate for the procedure, the surgery itself, risks, and what to expect after the procedure. This page is also available in Spanish.

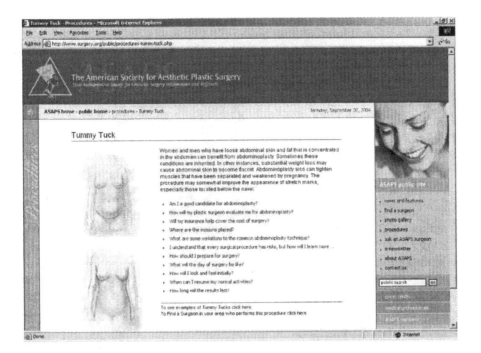

FIGURE 5.7. American Society for Aesthetic Plastic Surgery—Tummy Tuck <http://www.surgery.org/public/procedures-tummytuck.php> Reprinted with permission of American Society for Aesthetic Plastic Surgery.

American Society of Plastic Surgeons—Abdominoplasty (Tummy Tuck)
<http://www.plasticsurgery.org/public_education/procedures/Abdominoplasty.cfm>

The ASPS public information page on tummy tucks includes a description of the surgery, risks, postsurgical recovery, and before/after illustrations.

CosmeticSurgeryFYI.com—Abdominoplasty
<http://www.cosmeticsurgeryfyi.com/surgeries/abdominoplasty.html>

This site contains a general description about the tummy tuck procedure and who is a good candidate for the surgery. The site contains links to a photo gallery and before/after photos. The cosmetic surgeon locator service is limited to participating physicians. Spanish/German language information is available.

iEnhance—Abdominoplasty (Tummy Tuck)
<http://www.ienhance.com/procedure/default.asp>

Link directly to the "Procedures" page and select "Plastic Surgery," then, under "Abdomen" select "Abdominoplasty (Tummy Tuck)." This page includes basic information about tummy tucks, from the selection of patients and the surgical procedure to the risks, postsurgery, and costs.

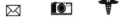

Medem—Surgery of the Abdomen: Abdominoplasty
<http://www.medem.com>

To get to the page on abdominoplasty, select "For Patients—Medical Library," and then select "Plastic Surgery/Cosmetic and Reconstructive Procedures," then "Other Cosmetic Procedures," and finally "Surgery of the Abdomen: Abdominoplasty." An alternate method is to input "tummy tuck" in the Search box on the main page, and then select from the choices that appear. The abdominoplasty page is produced by the American Society of Plastic Surgeons and duplicates the ASPS page.

Tuck That Tummy!
<http://www.tuckthattummy.com>

This site (see Figure 5.8) is produced by Enhancement Media, a company that has a group of "sister" sites on many cosmetic surgery topics. The site is easy to navigate, with links on the left-hand side that go to pages on "Your Anatomy," the surgical procedure, "Road to Recovery," selecting a surgeon, costs and financing, and more. Within each page are links to fairly extensive information; for example, the surgical procedure page in-

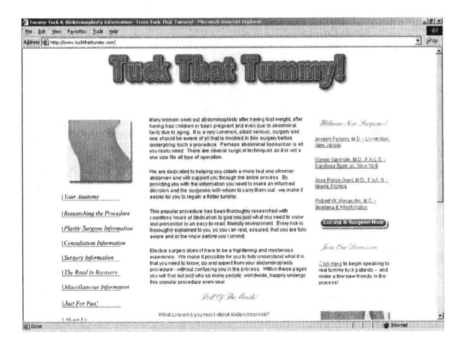

FIGURE 5.8. Tuck That Tummy!
<http://www.tuckthattummy.com>
Reprinted with permission of Enhancement Media.

cludes topics such as: "Preparing yourself emotionally" and an extensive description of the procedure with diagrams. Within "Plastic Surgeon Information" are links to help you research your surgeon (medical license, certifications, malpractice, etc.) and how to select a surgeon. The photo gallery is located under "Miscellaneous Information."

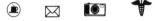

Tummy Tuck Resource
<http://www.tummy-tuck-resource.com>

This site bills itself as "a safety and resource site for abdominoplasty surgery." It includes photographs, risks, a description of the surgery, anesthesia, and what to expect following the procedure. "Find a Tummy Tuck Surgeon in Your Area," listed by state, appears on each page, but when you select a state and then your area within the state, only a form comes up to contact a doctor, without giving a doctor's name.

Yes They're Fake!—Abdominoplasty
<http://www.yestheyrefake.net/abdominoplasty.htm>

Go directly to the URL, or go to the main page <http://www. yestheyrefake.net>, select "Body Procedures," and then "Abdominoplasty." The page describes indications for the surgery and whether you are a good candidate for it (it is recommended that you wait until you are done having children), the types of procedures (types of incisions and endoscopic abdominoplasty to mini versus full abdominoplasty), risks and complications, and more.

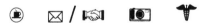

NOTE

1. "Lipoplasty." American Society of Plastic Surgeons. Available: <http://www. plasticsurgery.org/public_education/procedures/Lipoplasty.cfm>.

Chapter 6

Cosmetic Surgery of the Breast

Plastic surgery of the breast is usually performed for cosmetic purposes (e.g., breast enlargement and breast lift). It is also performed for reconstructive purposes, often following a mastectomy due to breast cancer. Interestingly, breast reduction is considered a "reconstructive" procedure, although it can be performed for cosmetic reasons (I can't help but think that a man decided it was reconstructive rather than cosmetic).

Year after year, cosmetic surgery of the breast consistently ranks as one of the top cosmetic procedures requested by women. It is also one of the most controversial procedures because of the materials used for breast implants. In the United States, implants are regulated by the Food and Drug Administration (FDA), which is listed later in this chapter. The FDA information should be *required reading* for any woman considering breast implants.

Some Internet sites are relevant to all types of plastic surgery of the breast, so a "General" section comes first, followed by specific procedures—breast enlargement, breast lift, breast reconstruction, and breast reduction.

BREAST—GENERAL

American Academy of Cosmetic Surgery—Breast Surgery
<http://www.cosmeticsurgery.org/procedures/breast_surgery.asp?
mn=pc>

Go directly to the URL, or select "Patient Center," then "Learn About a Cosmetic Procedure," then "Breast Surgery." This page contains basic information about breast augmentation, breast lift, and breast reduction.

Bermant Plastic and Cosmetic Surgery
<http://www.plasticsurgery4u.com>

This site is provided by Michael Bermant, MD, a board certified physician in plastic surgery, who practices near Richmond, VA. Although the site is not well organized, it contains a wealth of information. Scroll until you get to "Breast Sculpture" and then link to information on breast lift, breast reduction, and inverted nipple surgery. The site subscribes to the HONcode principles.

Breast Surgery FYI
<http://www.breastsurgeryfyi.com>

This is a special section of Cosmetic Surgery FYI, which gives extensive information about breast surgery, including breast augmentation, breast lift, breast reduction, breast reconstruction, and breast implants. Included is a description of the surgical procedure, who is a candidate for surgery, and risks. Contains links to before/after photos. The commercial aspect is evident with a link to the surgeon locator on each page, plus financing information.

iEnhance—Breast
<http://www.ienhance.com/procedure/default.asp>

Go directly to the "Procedures" page, select "Plastic Surgery," and you will find a section about breast surgery that includes links to pages on breast asymmetry, breast implant revision, breast reconstruction, inverted nipple repair, breast augmentation, breast lift, and breast reduction (see separate listings later in this chapter).

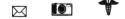

Imaginis.com—Cosmetic/Reconstructive Breast Surgery
<http://imaginis.com/breasthealth/menu-surgery.asp>

"Imaginis.com is dedicated to providing comprehensive information and service to improve and advance women's health." Billed as "the Breast Health Specialists," this site is a "comprehensive resource" for information about the breast and related women's health issues, covering topics such as breast cancer prevention, hormone replacement therapy, and ovarian cancer. The Cosmetic/Reconstructive Breast Surgery page (see Figure 6.1) leads to more specific pages that are listed in appropriate sections within this chapter. This site subscribes to the HONcode principles.

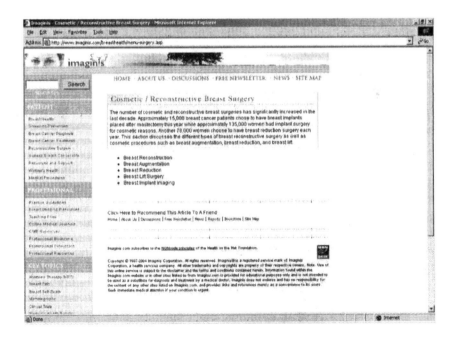

FIGURE 6.1. Imaginis—Cosmetic/Reconstructive Breast Surgery
<http://www.imaginis.com/breasthealth/menu-surgery.asp>
Reprinted with permission of Imaginis.

MedlinePlus—Breast Reconstruction
<http://www.nlm.nih.gov/medlineplus/breastreconstruction.html>

The Breast Reconstruction page of MedlinePlus (see Figure 6.2) brings together Internet resources dealing with breast implants, breast reduction, breast lift, and breast reconstruction following mastectomy. From information about risks and emotional aspects of the surgery to laws, statistics, and special conditions, this page is a great place to begin your search.

WebMD
<http://www.webmd.com>

WebMD is a general site that provides quality information on many topics. To find information on breast enlargement, breast implants, breast lift, and breast reduction, type any of these four topics into the search box and then choose the appropriate article from the list of "hits" that appears (not

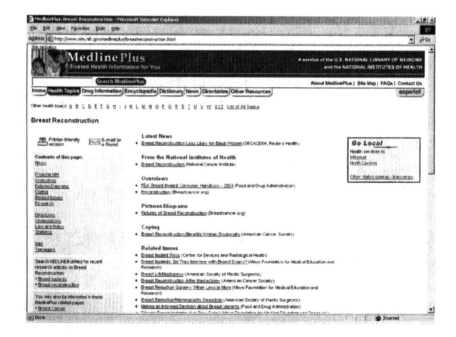

FIGURE 6.2. MedlinePlus—Breast Reconstruction
<http://www.nlm.nih.gov/medlineplus/breastreconstruction.html>

always the first choice; "breast reduction" was the second choice on the hit list at the time this site was reviewed).

BREAST ENLARGEMENT
(IMPLANTS, AUGMENTATION)

Breast enlargement is one of the most popular cosmetic surgery procedures for women, and, perhaps, the most controversial. Problems and complications resulting from (silicone) implants have led to regulation of breast implants in many countries (e.g., in the United States, the Center for Devices and Radiological Health of the U.S. Food and Drug Administration is the regulatory agency). Statistics are available both on breast augmentation (implants) and removal of breast implants. All procedures reported were conducted on women.

2003 statistics:

ASAPS:	254,140	(100 percent women)
ASPS:	280,401	(100 percent women)
	45,147 implant removals	(100 percent women)

American Society for Aesthetic Plastic Surgery—Breast Augmentation
<http://www.surgery.org/public/procedures-breastaug.php>

This ASAPS public page on breast augmentation (see Figure 6.3) is geared directly to women. This page leads to additional pages containing information about the surgical procedure, types of implants, risks, before-and-after surgery issues, and more. This is one of the better sites about breast augmentation. Included are illustrations and photos. This page is also available in Spanish.

American Society of Cosmetic Breast Surgery
<http://ascbs.org>

The ASCBS is a society dedicated to providing "the highest possible quality of care to women who wish to have cosmetic breast surgery." Infor-

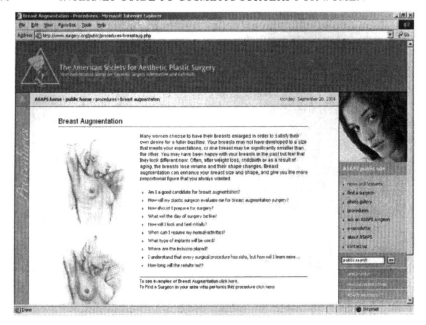

FIGURE 6.3. American Society for Aesthetic Plastic Surgery—Breast Augmentation
<http://www.surgery.org/public/procedures-breastaug.php>
Reprinted with permission of American Society for Aesthetic Plastic Surgery.

mation provided here is for breast augmentation surgery and includes photos, types of implants, a description of the surgery, problems/risks, and how to locate a surgeon.

**American Society of Plastic Surgeons—Breast Augmentation
<http://www.plasticsurgery.org/public_education/procedures/
AugmentationMammoplasty.cfm>**

The ASPS public information page on breast augmentation (augmentation mammoplasty) includes a description of the surgery, types of implants, risks, anesthesia, postsurgical recovery, and before/after illustrations (see Figure 6.4). Because of the required approval by the FDA for implant materials, it is especially important to read the ASPS press releases. Go to the main page and select "News Room" and "Press Releases"

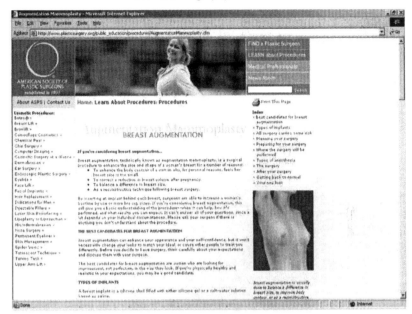

FIGURE 6.4. American Society of Plastic Surgeons—Breast Augmentation
<http://www.plasticsurgery.org/public_education/procedures/
AugmentationMammoplasty.cfm>
© 2004 American Society of Plastic Surgeons. All rights reserved. Learn more at
<www.plasticsurgery.org>.

or go directly to <http://www.plasticsurgery.org/news_room/press_
releases/index.cfm>. Releases include topics such as "ASPS Supports
FDA Regulatory Process Regarding Silicone Breast Implants" (1/8/04)
and "FDA Revises Silicone Implant Data Needs" (1/8/04). The "News
Room" also has a "Silicone Implants Press Kit" that groups information
together at <http://www.plasticsurgery.org/news_room/Silicone-Breast-
Implants-Press-Kit-Index.cfm>.

Breast Augmentation FYI
<http://www.breastaugmentationfyi.com>

A special section of Cosmetic Surgery FYI, this site gives extensive information about breast augmentation, including the surgical procedure,

who is a candidate for surgery, risks, and links to before/after photos. The commercial aspect is evident with a link to the surgeon locator on each page, plus financing information. You should also check out <http://www.breastsurgeryfyi.com>.

Breast Implants 4 You
<http://www.breastimplants4you.com>

This site is produced by Enhancement Media. The site is easy to navigate, with links that go to pages on anatomy, the surgical procedure, recovery, selecting a surgeon, costs and financing, and more. Within each page are links to fairly extensive information; for example, in "About Breast Augmentation" are topics covering breast-feeding after augmentation, risks and complications, silicone and saline-filled implants, and a photo gallery. Within "Plastic Surgeon Information" are links to help you research your surgeon (medical license, certifications, malpractice, etc.).

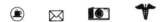

iEnhance—Breast Augmentation
<http://www.ienhance.com/procedure/default.asp>

Go directly to the "Procedures" page and select "Plastic Surgery," then under "Breast" select "Breast Augmentation." The page includes basic information such as patient selection, surgical procedure, risks, and post-surgical recovery. Also check out the page on "Breast Implant Revision."

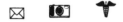

Imaginis—Breast Augmentation
<http://imaginis.com/breasthealth/augmentation.asp>

This Imaginis page overviews the initial consultation for breast augmentation, discusses the surgery and what will happen after the surgery, possible side effects, and breast-feeding following augmentation surgery. Links to additional resources are given.

Medicines and Healthcare Products Regulatory Agency
<http://www.medical-devices.gov.uk>

This is an executive agency of the Department of Health, United Kingdom. Select "Key Topics" and then "Breast Implants" to go to the U.K. Department of Health's main page about breast implants. Basic information about implants and cancer, complications, connective tissue disease, and types of breast implants is available. The United Kingdom operates a National Breast Implant Registry Web page (http://www.silicone-review.gov.uk/registry), which includes information about the agency and regulation of breast implants. Using the site's search feature, typing "breast implants" brings up a variety of regulatory news and safety warnings. This page is useful not only for U.K. residents, but for any woman considering breast implants.

U.S. Food and Drug Administration, Center for Devices and Radiological Health—Breast Implants
<http://www.fda.gov/cdrh/breastimplants/index.html>

The U.S. Food and Drug Administration (FDA), Center for Devices and Radiological Health, regulates breast implants. The site (see Figure 6.5) has a comprehensive "Breast Implant Consumer Handbook," an extensive (eighty-two-page) document in PDF format that covers everything from the surgery to risks, serious problems, and FDA regulatory activities related to breast implants (status/availability of implants); click on the link just under the "Handbook" (Breast Implants—An Information Update—2000), or go directly to <http://www.fda.gov/cdrh/breastimplants/indexbib.html>. Other information includes a brochure on risks, photographs of complications, and information on breast implant studies. You can sign up for the "Breast Implant Listserv" to receive a monthly update from the FDA on implants. This site is a "must visit" for any woman considering breast implants.

University of Iowa Plastic Surgery—Breast Augmentation
<http://www.surgery.uiowa.edu/surgery/plastic/baugment.html>

This page, from a university plastic surgery department, gives basic information about breast implants, the surgical procedure, recovery, complications, and risks.

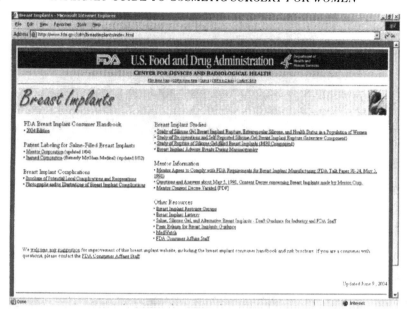

FIGURE 6.5. Breast Implant Consumer Handbook (FDA)
<http://www.fda.gov/cdrh/breastimplants/index.html>

Virtual Hospital—Breast Augmentation
<http://www.vh.org/adult/patient/surgery/plasticsurgery/breastaugmentation.html>

This page has brief but useful information about breast augmentation.

Yes They're Fake!—Breast Augmentation
<http://www.yestheyrefake.net/breast_augmentation_implants.html>

This site was created by a patient who has undergone cosmetic surgery herself. The page on breast augmentation can be located directly via the URL, or go to the main page <http://www.yestheyrefake.net>, select "Body Procedures," and then "Breast Augmentation." The page describes the surgery and types of implants used in the United States, breast-feeding after implants, risks, complications and contraindications of breast implants, a photo gallery, and more.

BREAST LIFT (MASTOPEXY)

A breast lift is used to lift and reshape sagging breasts. This procedure is reported exclusively for women.

2003 statistics:

ASAPS:	76,943	(100 percent women)
ASPS:	66,638	(100 percent women)

American Society for Aesthetic Plastic Surgery—Breast Lift
<http://www.surgery.org/public/procedures-breastlift.php>

This ASAPS public page on breast lifts (see Figure 6.6) is geared directly to women. This page leads to additional pages containing information about the surgical procedure, risks, before-and-after surgery issues, and more. This is one of the better sites about breast lifts. Contains illustrations and photos.

American Society of Plastic Surgeons—Breast Lift
<http://www.plasticsurgery.org/public_education/procedures/
Mastopexy.cfm>

This ASPS public information page on breast lifts (mastopexy) includes a description of the surgery, risks, anesthesia, postsurgical recovery, and before/after illustrations.

Breast Lift 4 You
<http://www.breastlift4you.com>

This site is produced by Enhancement Media. The site is easy to navigate, with links that go to pages on anatomy, the surgical procedure, recovery, selecting a surgeon, costs and financing, and more. Within each page are links to fairly extensive information; for example, in "Learn More About Breast Lift" are topics covering whether you are a candidate for a breast lift, various techniques and incision placements, risks and compli-

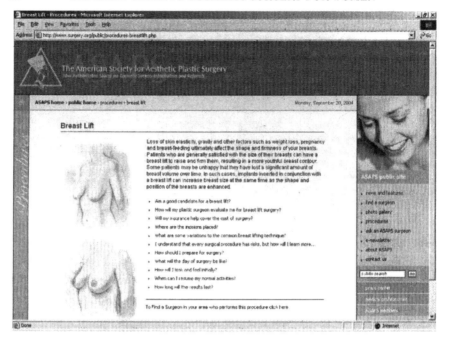

FIGURE 6.6. American Society for Aesthetic Plastic Surgery—Breast Lift
<http://www.surgery.org/public/procedures-breastlift.php>
Reprinted with permission of American Society for Aesthetic Plastic Surgery.

cations, and a photo gallery. Within "Plastic Surgeon Information" are
links to help you research your surgeon (medical license, certifications,
malpractice, etc.).

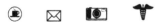

iEnhance—Breast Lift
<http://www.ienhance.com/procedure/default.asp>

Go directly to the "Procedures" page and select "Plastic Surgery," then
under "Breast" select "Breast Lift." The page includes basic information
such as patient selection, surgical procedure, risks, and postsurgical recovery.

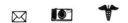

Imaginis—Breast Lift Surgery
<http://imaginis.com/breasthealth/breast_lift.asp>

This Imaginis page overviews the initial consultation for breast lift surgery, discusses the surgery and possible side effects. Links to additional resources are given.

Yes They're Fake!—Mastopexy
<http://www.yestheyrefake.net/breast_lift.htm>

This refreshingly candid site was created by a patient who has undergone cosmetic surgery herself. The page on breast lift (mastopexy) can be located directly via the URL, or go to the main page <http://www. yestheyrefake.net>, select "Body Procedures," and then "Breast Lift (Mastopexy)." The page describes the surgical options, risks, complications, contraindications, and more. You are referred to a sister site, Breast Lift 4 You <http://www.breastlift4you.com>, for more information. Also available is a page on the Benelli Mastopexy <http://www.yestheyrefake. net/benelli_mastopexy.htm>.

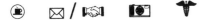

BREAST RECONSTRUCTION

Breast reconstruction is performed for many reasons, including reconstructive surgery following a mastectomy due to breast cancer. For this reason, many excellent resources are found on the Internet at cancer-related sites. Although breast reconstruction is considered a "plastic/reconstructive" procedure, it is included here because the result is considered by most to be cosmetic. Reconstruction of the breast restores a woman's self image both physically and mentally/emotionally.

2003 statistics:

ASPS: 68,521 breast reconstructions
        17,341 breast implant removals in reconstructive patients

American Cancer Society—Breast Reconstruction After Mastectomy
<http://www.cancer.org>

The American Cancer Society's page on "Breast Reconstruction After Mastectomy" is perhaps the best resource on the Internet concerning breast reconstruction. The URL is long, so the best way to locate it is to go to the ACS general page <http://www.cancer.org> and search the site using "breast reconstruction." This page covers everything from the types of procedures available for breast reconstruction (diagrams included) to questions to ask your plastic surgeon. Included are goals for reconstruction, when to have the surgery (immediate or delayed), an extensive glossary, and links to other resources. The site search will also locate other pages within the ACS site, such as "Post-Mastectomy Breast Reconstruction Complications Common" and "Breast Reconstruction Benefits Women Emotionally."

American Society of Plastic Surgeons—Breast Reconstruction (Following Breast Removal)
<http://www.plasticsurgery.org/public_education/procedures/ BreastReconstruction.cfm>

This ASAPS public page on breast reconstruction is geared directly to women who have had a breast removed due to cancer or another disease. This page contains information about the surgical options and procedures, risks, before-and-after surgery issues, and more. Contains illustrations and photos.

iEnhance—Breast Reconstruction
<http://www.ienhance.com/procedure/default.asp>

Go directly to the "Procedures" page and select "Plastic Surgery," then under "Breast" select "Breast Reconstruction." The page includes basic information for women requiring breast reconstruction, including patient selection, surgical procedures, risks, and postsurgical recovery, selecting a physician, and questions to ask your physician.

Imaginis—Breast Reconstruction
\<http://imaginis.com/breasthealth/reconstruction.asp\>

This page (see Figure 6.7) reviews the purpose of the surgery, types of breast reconstruction, complications of the surgery, advantages/disadvantages of having the surgery, and discusses issues such as questions to ask your physician (from the ACS), health insurance coverage, and breast imaging after your surgery. Links are available to other resources including the Imaginis page on "Breast Implant Screening" \<http://imaginis.com/breasthealth/breastimplant1.asp\>. You are referred to the ASPS to locate a plastic surgeon.

University of Iowa Plastic Surgery—Breast Reconstruction
\<http://www.surgery.uiowa.edu/surgery/plastic/brecon.html\>

This page, from a university plastic surgery department, gives basic information about breast reconstruction, including who should have the sur-

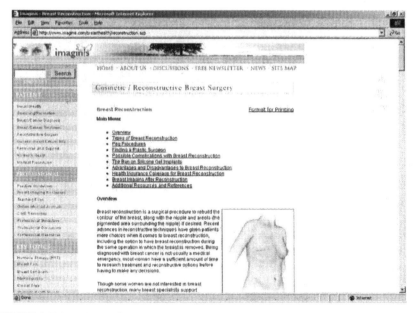

FIGURE 6.7. Imaginis—Breast Reconstruction
\<http://www.imaginis.com/breasthealth/reconstruction.asp\>
Reprinted with permission of Imaginis.

gery and timing for the procedure, techniques of breast reconstruction, and possible complications.

Virtual Hospital—Breast Reconstruction
<http://www.vh.org/adult/patient/surgery/plasticsurgery/
breastreconstruction.html>

This page includes information about who should have breast reconstruction, why and when they should have it, and surgical procedures that can be used.

BREAST REDUCTION

Reducing the size of a woman's breasts can help with medical problems caused by large breasts (e.g., back pain, breathing problems). Smaller breasts may be more proportionate to the woman's body. Breast reduction might be performed for cosmetic purposes, but many of the sites classify this surgery as a reconstructive procedure.

2003 statistics:

ASAPS:	147,173	(100 percent women)
ASPS:	113,140	(100 percent women)

American Society for Aesthetic Plastic Surgery—Breast Reduction
<http://www.surgery.org/public/procedures-breastreduce.php>

This ASAPS public page on breast reduction is geared directly to women. This page leads to additional pages containing information about the surgical procedure, risks, before-and-after surgery issues, and more. This is one of the better sites about breast reduction. Contains illustrations and photos. This page is also available in Spanish.

American Society of Plastic Surgeons—Breast Reduction
<http://www.plasticsurgery.org/public_education/procedures/ReductionMammaplasty.cfm>

This ASPS public information page on breast reduction (reduction mammaplasty) includes a description of the surgery, types of implants, risks, anesthesia, postsurgical recovery, and before/after illustrations. The ASPS places this procedure under "reconstructive" procedures. Also on the ASPS site, check out "BRAVO—Consumer's Guide to Breast Reduction" <http://www.plasticsurgery.org/public_education/BRAVO-Guide-to-Breast-Reduction.cfm>, available on the "Procedures" page under "Public Education." Links on this page go to state laws for breast reconstruction, FAQs, and patient experiences. BRAVO stands for Breast Reduction Assessment of Value and Outcomes, a study that was sponsored by the Plastic Surgery Educational Foundation.

Breast Reduction 4 You
<http://www.breastreduction4you.com>

This site (see Figure 6.8) is produced by Enhancement Media, a company that has a group of "sister" sites on many cosmetic surgery topics. The site is easy to navigate, with links that go to pages on anatomy, the surgical procedure, recovery, choosing a surgeon, costs and financing, etc. Within each page are links to fairly extensive information; for example, "Learning About Breast Reduction Surgery" covers topics regarding indications and contraindications for breast reduction, surgical techniques and incision placements, risks and complications, and more. Within "Plastic Surgeon Information" are links to help you research your surgeon (medical license, certifications, malpractice, etc.).

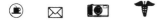

iEnhance—Breast Reduction
<http://www.ienhance.com/procedure/default.asp>

Go directly to the "Procedures" page and select "Plastic Surgery," then under "Breast" select "Breast Reduction." This page includes basic infor-

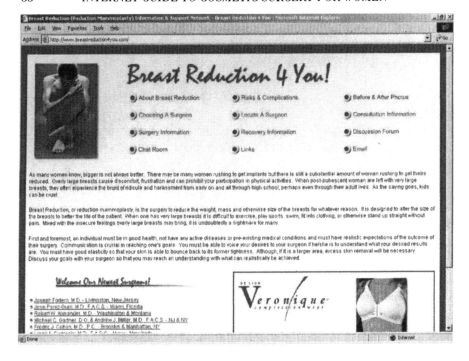

FIGURE 6.8. Breast Reduction 4 You
<http://www.breastreduction4you.com>
Reprinted with permission of Enhancement Media.

mation such as patient selection, surgical procedure, risks, and post-surgical recovery.

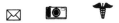

Imaginis—Breast Reduction
<http://imaginis.com/breasthealth/breast_reduction.asp>

This Imaginis page reviews the initial consultation for breast reduction, discusses the surgery and possible side effects, and breast-feeding following reduction surgery. Links to additional resources are given.

MayoClinic.com—Breast Reduction Surgery: When Less Is More
<http://www.mayoclinic.com/

Go to the general Mayo site and do a site search for "breast reduction." From the results, select "Breast Reduction Surgery: When Less Is More." This page gives excellent information on why the surgery is done and for whom, what happens before and during the surgery, recovery, and the benefits and risks.

U.S. Food and Drug Administration—Breast Reduction Often Good Medicine
<http://www.fda.gov/fdac/features/1997/197_brst.html>

This featured paper gives examples of women who have had breast reduction surgery (includes medical conditions and breast cancer), explains details of the surgery, post-op information, and adjusting to the difference after surgery.

University of Iowa Plastic Surgery—Breast Reduction
<http://www.surgery.uiowa.edu/surgery/plastic/breduc.html>

This page, from a university plastic surgery department, gives basic information about the surgical procedure, including planning and post-surgery.

Virtual Hospital—Breast Reduction
<http://www.vh.org/adult/patient/surgery/plasticsurgery/breastreduction.html>

This page from the Virtual Hospital has brief but useful information about breast reduction.

Yes They're Fake!—Breast Reduction
<http://www.yestheyrefake.net/breast_reduction.htm>

This refreshingly candid site was created by a patient who has undergone cosmetic surgery herself. The page on breast reduction can be located directly via the URL, or go to the main page <http://www.yestheyrefake. net>, select "Body Procedures," and then "Breast Reduction." The page discusses preoperative information, the surgery itself, what to expect in recovery, risks and complications, and more.

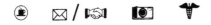

Chapter 7

Cosmetic Surgery
of the Face, Head, and Neck

This chapter covers cosmetic surgical procedures of the face, head, and neck. Hair transplantation can be found in Chapter 9. Nonsurgical cosmetic procedures involving primarily the skin, such as laser resurfacing and dermabrasion, can be found in Chapter 8, "Cosmetic Surgery of the Skin." Because there is an overlap with procedures involving the face and skin, cross-references will direct you to appropriate sections in this chapter or to other chapters. Those sites that either focus on the face, head, and neck, or have a special page that groups these procedures together, are listed in the "general" section. These sites may be listed again along with additional sites under individual procedures.

FACE, HEAD, AND NECK—GENERAL

American Academy of Facial Plastic and Reconstructive Surgery
<http://www.aafprs.org>

The AAFPRS Web site says "Trust Your Face to a Facial Plastic Surgeon." In the "Patients" section you'll find information about the society and an online magazine, but you will want to select "Procedures." From that page you can select the "Virtual Exam Room," which allows you to highlight the part of the face that you want surgery on, and then you can get information on the procedure. "Procedure Types" (see Figure 7.1) links you directly to information on facial surgical procedures that are online adaptations of the academy's brochures. FAQs includes some statistics on facial plastic surgery for women, while the glossary defines technical medical terms. This site also has a "Physician Finder."

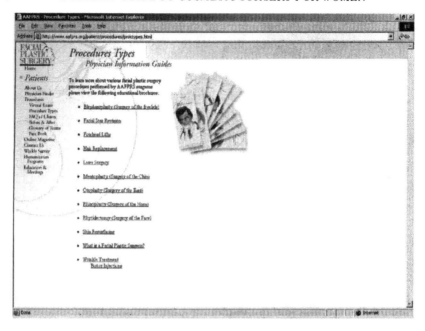

FIGURE 7.1. American Academy of Facial Plastic and Reconstructive Surgery—
Procedure Types
<http://aafprs.org/patient/procedures/proctypes.html>
Reprinted with permission of American Academy of Facial Plastic and Reconstructive
Surgery.

American Society of Ophthalmic Plastic and Reconstructive Surgery
<http://www.asoprs.org>

The American Society of Ophthalmic Plastic and Reconstructive Surgery is a membership organization of over 400 board certified ophthalmologists; this site serves both professionals and patients. Patient information available from this site includes surgery for drooping eyelids (blepharoplasty), laser skin resurfacing, cancer of the eyelids, and orbital trauma. Information is fairly brief, but does include before-and-after pictures. You are referred to your doctor for more information; the site has a physician directory searchable by state within the United States and over fourteen countries from around the world.

Facial Plastic Surgery Network
<http://www.facialplasticsurgery.net>

"The Facial Plastic Surgery Network is dedicated to helping you obtain solutions to your facial aesthetic concerns." This site is produced by Enhancement Media, a company that has a group of "sister" sites on many cosmetic surgery topics. The site is easy to navigate, with links at the top of the home page to "Facial Procedures," "Choosing a Surgeon," "Procedure FAQ," "Anesthesia Information," a photo gallery, chat groups and discussion forums, and more. A key page is "Facial Procedures," which has links to an extensive list of procedures (see Figure 7.2). Some of these are individually listed later in this chapter and also in Chapter 8, "Cosmetic Surgery of the Skin." Information is similar to the site Yes They're Fake! which is also produced by the same company.

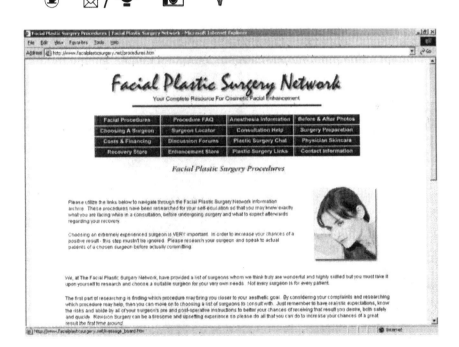

FIGURE 7.2. Facial Plastic Surgery Network—Facial Procedures
<http://www.facialplasticsurgery.net/procedures.htm>
Reprinted with permission of Enhancement Media.

iEnhance—Facial Plastic Surgery
<http://www.ienhance.com/speciality/facial.asp>

Go directly to the page (*sic*—speciality in URL), or begin at the general <http://www.ienhance.com> and select "Facial Plastic Surgery." This page has links to featured articles, archived articles, a photo gallery, a doctor locator, and specific surgical procedures. Select "Procedures" from this page, and then "Facial Plastic Surgery" to link to information on twenty-five to thirty facial plastic surgery procedures, from eyelid surgery to lip augmentation (see Figure 7.3). Also included here are skin procedures (see Chapter 8, "Cosmetic Surgery of the Skin") and hair transplantation (see Chapter 9, "Hair Transplantation for Women").

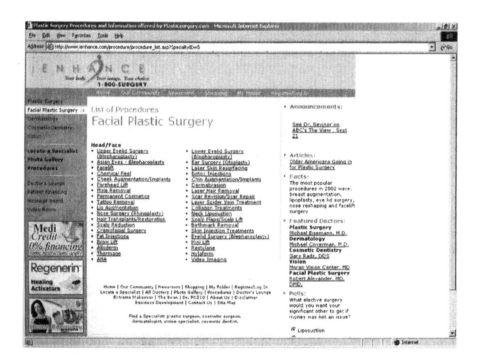

FIGURE 7.3. iEnhance—Facial Plastic Surgery List of Procedures
<http://www.ienhance.com/procedure/procedure_list.asp?SpecialtyID=5>
Reprinted with permission of iEnhance.com.

Medem—Procedures of the Face, Neck and Head
<http://www.medem.com/medlb/articleslb.cfm?sub_cat=2022>

The Medem page contains links to many facial cosmetic surgery procedures on the Medem site, for example, eyelid surgery, facelifts, facial implants, and facial scar revision. Information on the site is produced and made available to Medem by participating organizations (e.g., AAFPRS, ASPS, and AAO) and duplicates the material found at the Web sites of these organizations. Therefore, Medem is listed only in the "General" category for finding information, while the other organizations are listed as follows under specific procedures.

Yes They're Fake!—Facial Enhancement
<http://www.yestheyrefake.net/facial_plastic_surgery.html>

This is a refreshingly candid site, created by a patient who has undergone cosmetic surgery herself. Go directly to the URL, or go to the main page <http://www.yestheyrefake.net> and select "Facial Procedures." Many of the specific procedures from this "Facial Enhancement" page (see Figure 7.4) are listed later in this chapter (or in Chapter 8, "Cosmetic Surgery of the Skin") under the specific procedure, but it was not possible to list all. For those who want a more "formal" presentation, go to the Facial Plastic Surgery Network <http://www.facialplasticsurgery.net> for similar information.

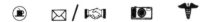

BLEPHAROPLASTY

See EYELID SURGERY (in this chapter).

BOTULINUM TOXIN (BOTOX) INJECTIONS

See Chapter 8, "Cosmetic Surgery of the Skin."

BROW LIFT

See FOREHEAD LIFT (in this chapter).

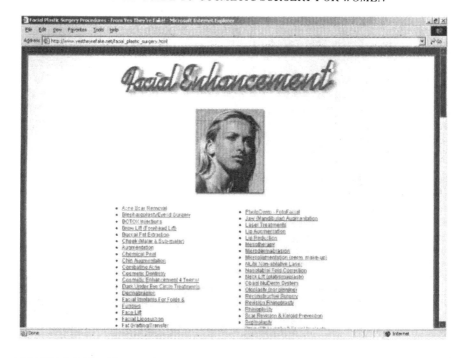

FIGURE 7.4. Yes They're Fake!—Facial Enhancement
<http://www.yestheyrefake.net/facial_plastic_surgery.html>
Reprinted with permission of Enhancement Media.

BUCCAL FAT PAD REMOVAL

This is the procedure to remove the fat pads in the lower cheeks to give a more defined look to the cheeks.

Facial Plastic Surgery Network—Buccal Fat Pad Extraction
<http://www.facialplasticsurgery.net/buccal_fat.htm>

This page can be reached directly via the URL, or go to the main page <http://www.facialplasticsurgery.net>, select "Facial Procedures," and then "Buccal Fat Extraction." This page is similar (procedure description, expectations, recovery, risks and complications, etc.) to Yes They're Fake! (see as follows), but without the informal, chatty comments.

Yes They're Fake!—Buccal Fat Pad Removal
<http://www.yestheyrefake.net/buccal_fat.htm>

This refreshingly candid site was created by a patient who has undergone cosmetic surgery herself. The page on buccal fat pad removal can be located directly via the URL, or go to the main page <http://www.yestheyrefake.net>, select "Facial Procedures," and then "Buccal Fat Pad Removal." The page describes the procedure (removing fat pads in the cheeks—"chipmunk cheeks"), whether you are a candidate for this surgery, the recovery, risks and complications, and more.

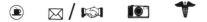

CHEEK IMPLANTS (AUGMENTATION)

See also FACIAL IMPLANTS (in this chapter).
Cheek implants are used to augment or increase the size of the cheek bones, giving a more defined look to the cheeks.

2003 statistics:

ASAPS:	8,287	(6,926 in women)
ASPS:	12,112	(9,759 in women)

All About Cheek Augmentation
<http://www.cheekaugmentation.com>

This site (see Figure 7.5) is produced by Enhancement Media and is part of the Facial Plastic Surgery network sites <http://www.facialplasticsurgery.net>. It is easy to navigate with links for "About Cheek Augmentation" (includes whether you are a candidate for the surgery, risks, complications, and photo gallery), "Your Options & More" (includes anesthesia and incision placement), "The Surgery," "Road to Recovery" (includes what to expect and complications), and more. Included in "Surgeon Information" are tips on how to choose a good surgeon and how to research the surgeon's credentials.

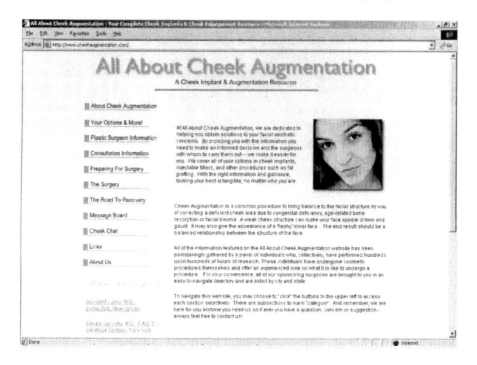

FIGURE 7.5. All About Cheek Augmentation
<http://www.cheekaugmentation.com>
Reprinted with permission of Enhancement Media.

American Academy of Cosmetic Surgery—Chin and Cheek Augmentation
<http://www.cosmeticsurgery.org/procedures/chin_and_cheek_augmentation.asp?mn=pc>

Go directly to the URL, or select "Patient Center," then "Learn About a Cosmetic Procedure," then "Chin and Cheek Augmentation." This page contains basic information about the procedure, postsurgery information, and risks. For costs, you are referred to your cosmetic surgeon.

iEnhance—Cheek Augmentation/Implants
\<http://www.ienhance.com/procedure/default.asp>

Link directly to the "Procedures" page and select either "Plastic Surgery" or "Facial Plastic Surgery," then under "Head/Face" select "Cheek Augmentation/Implants." Includes basic information such as patient selection, surgical procedure, risks, postsurgical recovery, and questions to ask your doctor.

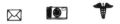

Yes They're Fake!—Cheek Augmentation
\<http://www.yestheyrefake.net/cheek_augmentation.htm>

This site was created by a patient who has undergone cosmetic surgery herself. The page on cheek augmentation can be located directly via the URL, or go to the main page \<http://www.yestheyrefake.net>, select "Facial Procedures," and then "Cheek Augmentation." The page helps you decide if you are a candidate for this surgery, lists surgical options and postsurgical recovery, and lists risks, complications, and contraindications. You are also referred to a "sister" site, All About Cheek Augmentation \<http://www.cheekaugmentation.com> (see previous listing), for more information.

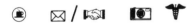

CHEEK REDUCTION

See BUCCAL FAT PAD REMOVAL (in this chapter).

CHEMICAL PEELS

See Chapter 8, "Cosmetic Surgery of the Skin."

CHIN AUGMENTATION (MENTOPLASTY)

Chin augmentation involves placing an implant over the bone and under the skin. This procedure is done for individuals who have a "weak" chin. By increasing the size of the chin, the face is given better balance and the profile is improved. Chin augmentation is often done in conjunction with nose surgery or facial liposuction.

2003 statistics:

ASAPS: 27,999 (21,118 in women)
ASPS: 16,306 (6,723 in women)

See also FACIAL IMPLANTS (in this chapter).

All About Chin Augmentation
<http://www.chinaugmentation.com>

This site is produced by Enhancement Media and is part of the Facial Plastic Surgery network sites <http://www.facialplasticsurgery.net>. It is easy to navigate with links for "About Chin Augmentation" (includes whether you are a candidate for the surgery, risks, complications, and photo gallery), "Your Options & More" (includes anesthesia and incision placement), "The Surgery," "Road to Recovery" (includes what to expect and complications), and more. Included in "Surgeon Information" are tips on how to choose a good surgeon and how to research the surgeon's credentials.

American Academy of Cosmetic Surgery—Chin and Cheek Augmentation
<http://www.cosmeticsurgery.org/procedures/chin_and_cheek_augmentation.asp?mn=mc>

Go directly to the URL, or select "Patient Center," then "Learn About a Cosmetic Procedure," then "Chin and Cheek Augmentation." This page contains basic information about both chin and cheek augmentation and postsurgery information; for risks and costs, you are referred to your cosmetic surgeon. This site also has a physician finder.

American Academy of Facial Plastic and Reconstructive Surgery— Understanding Mentoplasty Surgery
<http://www.aafprs.org/patient/procedures/mentoplasty.html>

The AAFPRS patient information includes a description of the procedure, deciding on chin surgery, postsurgery information, and before/after illustrations.

American Society of Plastic Surgeons—Chin Surgery
<http://www.plasticsurgery.org/public_education/procedures/ Mentoplasty.cfm>

The ASPS information page only has brief information about chin surgery. Check also the ASPS page on Facial Implants (Chin, Cheeks & Jaw Surgery) <http://www.plasticsurgery.org/public_education/procedures/ FacialImplants.cfm>.

iEnhance—Chin Augmentation/Implants
<http://www.ienhance.com/procedure/default.asp>

Link directly to the "Procedures" page and select either "Plastic Surgery" or "Facial Plastic Surgery," then under "Head/Face" select "Chin Augmentation/Implants." The page includes basic information such as patient selection, surgical procedure, risks, postsurgical recovery, and questions to ask your doctor.

Yes They're Fake!—Chin Augmentation
<http://www.yestheyrefake.net/chin_augmentation.htm>

The page on chin augmentation can be located directly via the URL, or go to the main page <http://www.yestheyrefake.net>, select "Facial Procedures," and then "Chin Augmentation." The page helps you decide if you are a candidate for chin surgery, lists surgical options and postsurgical recovery, and lists risks, complications, and contraindications. You are also referred to a "sister" site, All About Chin Augmentation <http://www. chinaugmentation.com> (see previous listing), for more information.

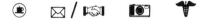

DERMABRASION

See Chapter 8, "Cosmetic Surgery of the Skin."

EAR SURGERY (OTOPLASTY)

Otoplasty is the surgical procedure used to correct ears that protrude, or stick out from the side of the head, or to reduce the size of the ears. Commonly called "pinning back" the ears, otoplasty improves one's appearance without affecting hearing.

2003 statistics:

ASAPS:	27,814	(15,298 in women)
ASPS:	26,612	(15,133 in women)

American Academy of Cosmetic Surgery—Otoplasty (Ear Surgery) <http://www.cosmeticsurgery.org/procedures/otoplasty__ear_ surgery_.asp?mn=pc>

Go directly to the URL, or select "Patient Center," then "Learn About a Cosmetic Procedure," then "Otoplasty (Ear Surgery)." The page contains basic information about the procedure, postsurgery information, and risks. For costs, you are referred to your cosmetic surgeon.

American Academy of Facial Plastic and Reconstructive Surgery— Understanding Otoplasty Surgery <http://www.aafprs.org/patient/procedures/otoplasty.html>

The AAFPRS patient information includes a description of the procedure, deciding on ear surgery, and postsurgery information, and also includes illustrations.

American Academy of Otolaryngology—Head and Neck Surgery— Plastic Surgery of the Ear
<http://www.entnet.org/healthinfo/ears/plastic_surgery.cfm>

The AAO-HNS page discusses pinning back the ears, correcting ear deformities, and torn earlobes.

American Society of Plastic Surgeons—Otoplasty (Ear Surgery)
<http://www.plasticsurgery.org/public_education/procedures/ otoplasty.cfm>

The ASPS public information page on ear surgery includes a description of the surgery, anesthesia, risks, postsurgical recovery, and before/ after illustrations.

Bermant Plastic and Cosmetic Surgery—Otoplasty Cosmetic Sculpture of the Ears
<http://www.plasticsurgery4u.com>

This site is provided by Dr. Michael Bermant, a board certified physician in plastic surgery, who practices near Richmond, VA. Although the site is not well organized, it contains a wealth of information. Scroll until you get to "Ear Sculpture" and then link to information about otoplasty. The site subscribes to the HONcode.

Facial Plastic Surgery Network—Otoplasty (Ear Pinning, Reshaping)
<http://www.facialplasticsurgery.net/otoplasty.htm>

This page can be reached directly via the URL, or go to the main page <http://www.facialplasticsurgery.net>, select "Facial Procedures," and then "Otoplasty (Ear Pinning)." This page is similar (whether you are a candidate for surgery, procedure description, expectations, recovery, risks and complications, etc.) to Yes They're Fake! (see as follows), but without the informal, chatty comments.

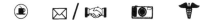

iEnhance—Ear Surgery (Otoplasty)
<http://www.ienhance.com/procedure/default.asp>

Go directly to the "Procedures" page and select either "Plastic Surgery" or "Facial Plastic Surgery," then under "Head/Face" select "Ear Surgery (Otoplasty)." This page includes basic information such as patient selection, surgical procedure, risks, postsurgical recovery, and questions to ask your doctor.

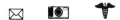

MedicineNet.com—Cosmetic/Reconstructive Surgery of the Ear (Otoplasty) Surgical Instructions
<http://www.medicinenet.com/otoplasty/article.htm>

This article describes the surgical procedure, including what happens before, during, and after surgery, plus risks and complications. "MedicineNet, Inc. is an online, healthcare media publishing company" that subscribes to the HONcode.

University of Iowa Plastic Surgery—Otoplasty
<http://www.surgery.uiowa.edu/surgery/plastic/otoplst.html>

This page, from a university plastic surgery department, describes the development of the ears, the reasons for having otoplasty, the procedure, and risks and complications. Photos are included.

Yes They're Fake!—Otoplasty
<http://www.yestheyrefake.net/otoplasty.htm>

This is a refreshingly candid site, created by a patient who has undergone cosmetic surgery herself. The page on otoplasty can be located directly via the URL, or go to the main page <http://www.yestheyrefake. net>, select "Facial Procedures," and then "Otoplasty." The page helps you decide if you are a candidate for otoplasty (which is described here as ear pinning), describes preparing for surgery, the surgical procedure, post-surgical recovery, and lists risks and complications.

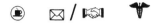

EYELID SURGERY (BLEPHAROPLASTY)

Blepharoplasty is cosmetic surgery of the eyelids. It removes the excess fat from the upper and lower eyelids. The procedure corrects droopy eyelids and can remove the "bags" from under your eyes. Blepharoplasty is often done with other cosmetic surgery of the face, such as a facelift or skin resurfacing.

2003 statistics:

ASAPS:	267,627	(216,829 in women)
ASPS:	246,633	(200,324 in women)

American Academy of Facial Plastic and Reconstructive Surgery—Understanding Blepharoplasty
<http://www.aafprs.org/patient/procedures/blepharoplasty.html>

The AAFPRS site discusses making the decision to have blepharoplasty, the surgery, and what to expect postsurgery. Before/after illustrations are included.

American Society for Aesthetic Plastic Surgery—Eyelid Surgery
<http://www.surgery.org/public/procedures-eyelid.php>

This ASAPS public page on eyelid surgery leads to additional pages containing information about the surgical procedure, risks, before and after surgery, and more. This is one of the better sites available about eyelid surgery.

American Society for Dermatologic Surgery—Aging Eyelids
<http://www.asds.net/Patients/FactSheets/patients-Fact_Sheet-aging_eyelids.html>

Go directly to the URL, or select "Patients," then "Fact Sheets," and then "Aging Eyelids." This ASDS fact sheet about aging eyelids describes blepharoplasty, including information about the procedure, postoperative effects, and complications.

American Society of Ophthalmic Plastic and Reconstructive
Surgery—Blepharoplasty
<http://www.asoprs.org/Pages/blepharoplasty.html>

This site includes basic information about cosmetic surgery of the eyelids. Additional information about eyelid drooping is also available from the "Patient" page <http://www.asoprs.org/Pages/Patients.html>.

American Society of Plastic Surgeons—Blepharoplasty (Eyelids)
<http://www.plasticsurgery.org/public_education/procedures/Blepharoplasty.cfm>

The ASPS public information page on eyelid surgery includes a description of the surgery, anesthesia, risks, postsurgical recovery, and before/after illustrations. This page is available in Spanish (choose Spanish from Procedures page or go directly to <http://www.plasticsurgery.org/public_education/procedures/Blefaroplastia.cfm>).

Bermant Plastic and Cosmetic Surgery
<http://www.plasticsurgery4u.com>

This site is provided by Dr. Michael Bermant, a board certified physician in plastic surgery, who practices near Richmond, VA. Although the site is not well organized, it contains a wealth of information. Scroll until you get to "Eyelid Sculpture" and then link to information about blepharoplasty. The site subscribes to the HONcode principles.

Facial Plastic Surgery Network—Blepharoplasty: Eyelid Tuck Surgery
<http://www.facialplasticsurgery.net/blepharoplasty.htm>

This page can be reached directly via the URL, or go to the main page <http://www.facialplasticsurgery.net>, select "Facial Procedures," and then "Blepharoplasty." This page is similar (procedure description, expectations, recovery, risks and complications, etc.) to Yes They're Fake! (see as follows), but without the informal, chatty comments.

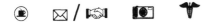

iEnhance—Eyelid Surgery (Blepharoplasty)
<http://www.ienhance.com/procedure/default.asp>

Go directly to the "Procedures" page and select either "Plastic Surgery" or "Facial Plastic Surgery," then, under "Head/Face" are four separate pages: "Upper Eyelid Surgery," "Lower Eyelid Surgery," "Blepharoplasty (Eyelid Surgery)," and "Asian Eyes-Blepharoplasty." The general blepharoplasty page has little information, but the other three pages include basic information such as patient selection, surgical procedure, risks, post-surgical recovery, and questions to ask your doctor.

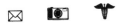

University of Iowa Plastic Surgery—Plastic Surgery of the Eyes
<http://www.surgery.uiowa.edu/surgery/plastic/bleph.html>

This page, from a university plastic surgery department, gives basic information about eyelid surgery.

Virtual Hospital—Blepharoplasty
<http://www.vh.org/adult/patient/surgery/plasticsurgery/ blepharoplasty.html>

This page from the Virtual Hospital has brief but useful information about surgery of the eyelids or eyebrows.

Yes They're Fake!—Blepharoplasty
<http://www.yestheyrefake.net/blepharoplasty.htm>

This is a refreshingly candid site, created by a patient who has undergone cosmetic surgery herself. The page on blepharoplasty can be located directly via the URL, or go to the main page <http://www.yestheyrefake. net>, select "Facial Procedures," and then "Blepharoplasty/Eyelid Surgery." The page helps you decide if you are a candidate for blepharoplasty (eyelid surgery or eyelid lift), describes preparing for surgery, the surgical procedure, and postsurgical recovery, and lists risks and complications.

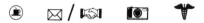

FACELIFT (RHYTIDECTOMY)

Rhytidectomy is the technical name for a facelift. Facelifts are performed to reduce the effects of aging by removing wrinkles that form in the skin, along with the removal of excess fat and tightening of the muscles. Facelifts are often performed along with eyelid surgery, a forehead lift, and other facial cosmetic procedures.

2003 statistics:

ASAPS:	125,581	(112,025 in women)
ASPS:	128,667	(115,908 in women)

American Academy of Cosmetic Surgery—Rhytidectomy (Facelift)
<http://www.cosmeticsurgery.org/procedures/rhytidectomy_face_ lift_.asp?mn=pc>

Go directly to the URL, or select "Patient Center," then "Learn About a Cosmetic Procedure," then "Rhytidectomy (Facelift)." The page contains basic information about the facelift procedure, pre- and postsurgery information, and risks.

American Academy of Facial Plastic and Reconstructive Surgery—Understanding Rhytidectomy
<http://www.aafprs.org/patient/procedures/rhytidectomy.html>

The AAFPRS patient information includes a description of the procedure, deciding on a facelift, and postsurgery information, and also includes before/after illustrations.

American Society for Aesthetic Plastic Surgery—Facelift
<http://www.surgery.org/public/procedures-facelift.php>

The ASAPS public page on facelift surgery leads to additional pages containing information about the surgical procedure, risks, before and after surgery, and more. This is one of the better sites available about facelift surgery.

American Society of Plastic Surgeons—Rhytidectomy (Facelift)
<http://www.plasticsurgery.org/public_education/procedures/rhytidectomy.cfm>

This ASPS public information page on facelift includes a description of the surgery, anesthesia, risks, postsurgical recovery, and before/after illustrations. This page is available in Spanish (choose Spanish from Procedures page or go directly to <http://www.plasticsurgery.org/public_education/procedures/Ritidectomia.cfm>).

Bermant Plastic and Cosmetic Surgery
\<http://www.plasticsurgery4u.com\>

This site is provided by Dr. Michael Bermant, a board certified physician in plastic surgery, who practices near Richmond, VA. Although the site is not well organized, it contains a wealth of information. Scroll until you get to "Facial Sculpture," which is primarily about facelifts. Links go to pages on facelift, neck lift, and brow lift. The site subscribes to the HONcode principles.

Facelift FYI
\<http://www.faceliftfyi.com\>

A special section of the Cosmetic Surgery FYI site, this site gives extensive information about facelifts, including the surgical procedure, who is a candidate for surgery, and risks. The site contains links to before/after photos. The commercial aspect is evident with a link to the surgeon locator on each page, plus financing information.

Facial Plastic Surgery Network—Face Lift
\<http://www.facialplasticsurgery.net/face_lift.htm\>

This page can be reached directly via the URL, or go to the main page \<http://www.facialplasticsurgery.net\>, select "Facial Procedures," and then "Face Lift." This page is similar (types of facelift, procedure description, expectations, recovery, risks and complications, etc.) to Yes They're Fake! (see as follows).

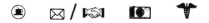

iEnhance—Face Lift
\<http://www.ienhance.com/procedure/default.asp\>

Go directly to the "Procedures" page and select either "Plastic Surgery" or "Facial Plastic Surgery," then under "Head/Face" select "Face Lift." The page includes basic information such as patient selection, surgical procedure, risks, postsurgical recovery, and questions to ask your doctor.

MayoClinic.com—Saving Face: The Nips and Tucks of Face-Lifts
<http://www.mayoclinic.com/>

Go to the general Mayo site and do a site search for "face lift" to locate the page on "Saving Face." This page cautions prospective patients to have a realistic expectation of results, describes the procedure and postsurgical effects, along with complications.

University of Iowa Plastic Surgery—Facelift
<http://www.surgery.uiowa.edu/surgery/plastic/flift.html>

This page, from a university plastic surgery department, gives basic information about facelifts, what to expect postsurgery, and complications.

Virtual Hospital—Facelifts: Frequently Asked Questions
<http://www.vh.org/adult/patient/surgery/plasticsurgery/facelift.
html>

This page from the Virtual Hospital has information about facelifts, presented as a question and answer session with Dr. Al Aly, of the University of Iowa Hospitals and Clinics.

Yes They're Fake!—Face Lift
<http://www.yestheyrefake.net/face_lift.htm>

This is a refreshingly candid site, created by a patient who has undergone cosmetic surgery herself. The page on facelifts can be located directly via the URL, or go to the main page <http://www.yestheyrefake.net>, select "Facial Procedures," and then "Face Lift." The page describes the underlying facial structure, whether you are a candidate for a facelift, the types of facelifts, preparing for surgery and the recovery, risks, and complications, questions to ask, and more. Also check out the link to "Feather Life (APTOS Threads)" from the "Facial Procedures" page, or go directly to <http://www.yestheyrefake.net/feather_lift.htm>.

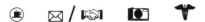

FACIAL IMPLANTS

Facial implants alter and enhance the shape of your face, and are most commonly performed on the cheekbones and chin (*see also* CHEEK IMPLANTS, CHIN AUGMENTATION, and JAW AUGMENTATION in this chapter). The implants may be done in conjunction with other cosmetic procedures of the face, such as facelifts or rhinoplasty (surgery of the nose).

2003 statistics:

ASAPS: 8,287 cheek implants (6,926 in women)
ASPS: 12,112 cheek implants (9,759 in women)

American Academy of Cosmetic Surgery—Chin and Cheek Augmentation
<http://www.cosmeticsurgery.org/procedures/chin_and_cheek_augmentation.asp?mn=pc>

Go directly to the URL, or select "Patient Center," then "Learn About a Cosmetic Procedure," then "Chin and Cheek Augmentation." The page contains basic information about the procedure, postsurgery information, and risks. For costs, you are referred to your cosmetic surgeon.

American Society for Aesthetic Plastic Surgery—Facial Implants
<http://www.surgery.org/public/procedures-faceimplants.php>

This ASAPS public page on facial implants describes the surgical technique, benefits, and risks of facial implants.

American Society of Plastic Surgeons—Facial Implants (Chin, Cheeks & Jaw Surgery)
<http://www.plasticsurgery.org/public_education/procedures/facialimplants.cfm>

The ASPS public information page on facial implants (see Figure 7.6) includes a description of the surgery, anesthesia, risks, postsurgical recov-

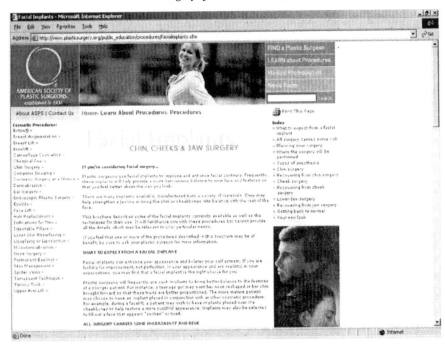

FIGURE 7.6. American Society of Plastic Surgeons—Facial Implants (Chin, Cheeks & Jaw Surgery)
<http://www.plasticsurgery.org/public_education/procedures/facialimplants.cfm>
© 2004 American Society of Plastic Surgeons. All rights reserved. Learn more at <www.plasticsurgery.org>.

ery, and before/after illustrations. Chin, cheek, and lower jaw surgery procedures are discussed.

Virtual Hospital—Facial Implants: Frequently Asked Questions
<http://www.vh.org/adult/patient/surgery/plasticsurgery/facialimplants.html>

This page from the Virtual Hospital has information about facial implants, presented as a question and answer session with Dr. Al Aly, of the University of Iowa Hospitals and Clinics.

Yes They're Fake!—Facial Implants
\<http://www.yestheyrefake.net/facial_implants.htm\>

This is a refreshingly candid site, created by a patient who has undergone cosmetic surgery herself. The page on facial implants can be located directly via the URL, or go to the main page \<http://www.yestheyrefake. net\>, select "Facial Procedures," and then "Facial Implants." The page primarily discusses five implant products: Advanta Facial Implant, Gore-Tex Facial Implant, Gore-Tex Strands and Multi-Strands, SoftForm, and UltraSoft.

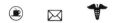

FACIAL LIPOSUCTION

Facial liposuction is the removal of fat from the face and under the chin. The procedure is done to give a more defined look to the face and can be performed in conjunction with other procedures such as a chin implant.

Facial Plastic Surgery Network—Facial & Submental Liposuction
\<http://www.facialplasticsurgery.net/facial_liposuction.htm\>

This page can be reached directly via the URL, or go to the main page \<http://www.facialplasticsurgery.net\>, select "Facial Procedures," and then "Facial Liposuction." This page is similar (whether you are a candidate for surgery, procedure description, expectations, recovery, risks, and complications, etc.) to Yes They're Fake! (see as follows).

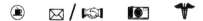

Yes They're Fake!—Facial Liposuction
\<http://www.yestheyrefake.net/facial_liposuction.htm\>

This is a refreshingly candid site, created by a patient who has undergone cosmetic surgery herself. The page on facial liposuction can be located directly via the URL, or go to the main page \<http://www. yestheyrefake.net\>, select "Facial Procedures," and then "Facial Liposuction." The page helps you decide if you are a candidate for facial liposuction surgery, describes the preoperative preparation, the surgery, post-surgical recovery, and lists risks and complications.

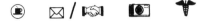

FAT INJECTIONS

See FAT INJECTIONS in Chapter 8, "Cosmetic Surgery of the Skin."

FOREHEAD LIFT (BROW LIFT)

A forehead (brow) lift is done to reduce the signs of aging in this area of the face. In the procedure, wrinkles are reduced/eliminated by removing excess skin and, if necessary, part of the underlying muscles. This procedure is frequently done with a facelift and/or eye surgery.

2003 statistics:

ASAPS: 76,696   (65,412 in women)
ASPS: 57,771   (49,290 in women)

American Academy of Cosmetic Surgery—Forehead Lift
<http://www.cosmeticsurgery.org/procedures/forehead_lift.asp?
mn=pc>

Go directly to the URL, or select "Patient Center," then "Learn About a Cosmetic Procedure," then "Forehead Lift." The page contains basic information about the surgical procedure for a forehead lift and postsurgery information.

American Academy of Facial Plastic and Reconstructive Surgery— Understanding Forehead and Brow Lift Surgery
<http://www.aafprs.org/patient/procedures/forehead_lifts.html>

The AAFPRS patient information includes a description of the procedure, deciding on forehead/brow lift surgery, and postsurgery information; it also includes before/after illustrations.

American Society for Aesthetic Plastic Surgery—Forehead Lift
<http://www.surgery.org/public/procedures-forehead.php>

This is the ASAPS public page on forehead lift (see Figure 7.7); it leads to additional pages containing information about the surgical procedure, risks, before and after surgery, and more. This is one of the better sites available about forehead lifts.

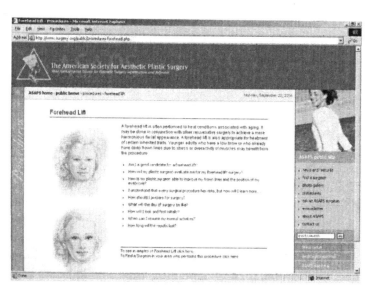

FIGURE 7.7. American Society for Aesthetic Plastic Surgery—Forehead Lift
<http://www.surgery.org/public/procedures-forehead.php>
Reprinted with permission of the American Society for Aesthetic Plastic Surgery.

American Society of Plastic Surgeons—Browlift (Forehead Lift)
<http://www.plasticsurgery.org/public_education/procedures/
  browlift.cfm>

This ASPS public information page on surgery of the forehead includes a description of the surgery, anesthesia, risks, postsurgical recovery, and before/after illustrations.

Bermant Plastic and Cosmetic Surgery—Brow Lift (Forehead Lift)
<http://www.plasticsurgery4u.com>

This site is provided by Dr. Michael Bermant, a board certified physician in plastic surgery, who practices near Richmond, Virginia. Although the site is not well organized, it contains a wealth of information. Scroll until you get to the single line—"Brow Lift the Surgery," and then link to the page on brow lifts. The site subscribes to the HONcode.

Facial Plastic Surgery Network—Forehead and Brow Lift Surgery
<http://www.facialplasticsurgery.net/brow_forehead_lift.htm>

This page can be reached directly via the URL, or go to the main page <http://www.facialplasticsurgery.net>, select "Facial Procedures," and then "Brow or Forehead Lift." This page is similar (procedure description, expectations, recovery, risks and complications, etc.) to Yes They're Fake! (see as follows), but without the informal, chatty comments.

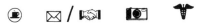

iEnhance—Forehead Lift
<http://www.ienhance.com/procedure/default.asp>

Go directly to the "Procedures" page and select either "Plastic Surgery" or "Facial Plastic Surgery," then under "Head/Face" select "Forehead Lift." The page includes basic information such as patient selection, surgical procedure (conventional and endoscopic forehead lift), risks, postsurgical recovery, and questions to ask your doctor.

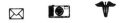

University of Iowa Plastic Surgery—Browlift
<http://www.surgery.uiowa.edu/surgery/plastic/browlift.html>

This page, from a university plastic surgery department, gives basic information about forehead surgery, what to expect postsurgery, and complications.

Virtual Hospital—Browlift
**<http://www.vh.org/adult/patient/surgery/plasticsurgery/browlift.
html>**

This page from the Virtual Hospital has brief but useful information about brow lifts.

Yes They're Fake!—Brow or Forehead Lift
<http://www.yestheyrefake.net/brow_lift.htm>

This is a refreshingly candid site, created by a patient who has undergone cosmetic surgery herself. The page on brow/forehead lift can be located directly via the URL, or go to the main page <http://www.
yestheyrefake.net>, select "Facial Procedures," and then "Brow Lift." The page helps you decide if you are a candidate for brow lift, describes the preoperative preparation, the surgery, and postsurgical recovery, and lists risks and complications.

⍟   ⊠ / ☜   📷   ⚕

JAW AUGMENTATION

Jaw augmentation is the cosmetic procedure that increases the size of the jaw (mandible), using a synthetic product. It can be done in conjunction with a chin implant, and also with nose surgery, to give a more balanced look to the face. *See also* FACIAL IMPLANTS (in this chapter).

All About Jaw Augmentation
<http://www.jawaugmentation.com>

This site is produced by Enhancement Media and is part of the Facial Plastic Surgery network sites <http://www.facialplasticsurgery.net>. It is easy to navigate with links on the left-hand side for "About Jaw Augmentation" (includes whether you are a candidate for the surgery, risks, complications, and photo gallery), "Your Options & More" (includes anesthesia and incision placement), "The Surgery," "Road to Recovery" (includes what to expect and complications), and more. Included in "Surgeon Information" are tips on how to choose a good surgeon and how to research the surgeon's credentials.

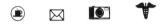

Facial Plastic Surgery Network—Jaw Augmentation & Jaw Implants
<http://www.facialplasticsurgery.net/jaw_augmentation.htm>

This page can be reached directly via the URL, or go to the main page <http://www.facialplasticsurgery.net>, select "Facial Procedures," and then "Jaw Augmentation." The page helps you decide if you are a candidate for chin surgery, lists surgical options and postsurgical recovery, and lists risks, complications, and contraindications, similar to Yes They're Fake! You are also referred to a "sister" site, All About Jaw Augmentation <http://www.jawaugmentation.com> (see previous listing), for more information.

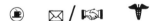

Yes They're Fake!—Jaw Augmentation
<http://www.yestheyrefake.net/jaw_augmentation.htm>

This is a refreshingly candid site, created by a patient who has undergone cosmetic surgery herself. The page on jaw augmentation can be located directly via the URL, or go to the main page <http://www.yestheyrefake.net>, select "Facial Procedures," and then "Jaw Augmentation." The page helps you decide if you are a candidate for jaw surgery, lists surgical options, postsurgical recovery, and risks, complications, and contraindications. You are also referred to a "sister" site, All About Jaw Augmentation <http://www.jawaugmentation.com> (see previous), for more information.

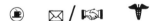

LASER SKIN RESURFACING

See CHEMICAL PEELS, DERMABRASION, and LASER SKIN RESURFAC-ING in Chapter 8, "Cosmetic Surgery of the Skin."

LIP AUGMENTATION

See also INJECTABLE FILLERS in Chapter 8, "Cosmetic Surgery of the Skin."

Lip augmentation increases the size of your lips. This procedure involves inserting a synthetic filler or injecting natural materials, and is used to augment the size of the lips for women with naturally thin lips, or to battle the signs of aging. Upper, lower, or both lips can be augmented.

2003 statistics:

ASAPS:	23,164	(22,722 in women)
	(other than injectable material)	
ASPS:	22,667	(21,478 in women)
	(other than injectable material)	

All About Lip Augmentation
<http://www.lipaugmentation.com>

This site (see Figure 7.8) is produced by Enhancement Media and is part of the Facial Plastic Surgery network sites <http://www.facialplasticsurgery. net>. It is easy to navigate with links to "Understanding Your Lips" (includes anatomy), "About Lip Augmentation" (includes whether you are a candidate for the surgery, risks, complications, and photo gallery), "Your Options and More" (includes anesthesia and incision placement), "Procedure Information," "Road to Recovery" (includes what to expect and complications), and more. Included in "Surgeon Information" are tips on how to choose a good surgeon and how to research the surgeon's credentials.

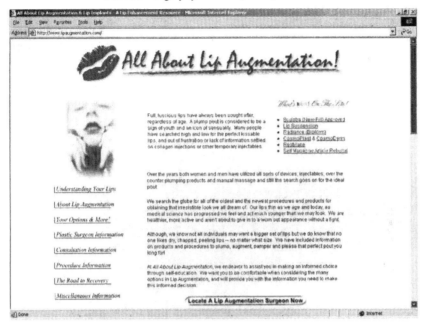

FIGURE 7.8. All About Lip Augmentation Home Page
<http://www.lipaugmentation.com>
Reprinted with permission of Enhancement Media.

American Society for Aesthetic Plastic Surgery—Lip Augmentation
<http://www.surgery.org/public/procedures-lipaug.php>

The ASAPS public page on lip augmentation contains general information about the procedure, a description of the technique, options to consider, benefits, and other considerations.

iEnhance—Lip Augmentation
<http://www.ienhance.com/procedure/default.asp>

Go directly to the "Procedures" page and select either "Plastic Surgery" or "Facial Plastic Surgery," then under "Head/Face" select "Lip Augmentation." The page includes basic information such as patient selection, surgical procedure, risks, postsurgical recovery, and questions to ask your doctor.

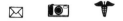

Yes They're Fake!—Lip Augmentation
<http://www.yestheyrefake.net/lip_augmentation.html>

This is a refreshingly candid site, created by a patient who has undergone cosmetic surgery herself. The page on lip augmentation can be located directly via the URL, or go to the main page <http://www.yestheyrefake.net>, select "Facial Procedures," and then "Lip Augmentation." The page helps you decide if you are a candidate for lip surgery, lists surgical options, postsurgical recovery, and risks, complications, and contraindications. You are also referred to a "sister" site, All About Lip Augmentation <http://www.lipaugmentation.com> (see previous), for more information.

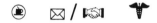

LIP REDUCTION

Lip reduction can be done for patients who feel that their lips are too large and wish to reduce their size. The procedure involves removing tissue from the lips (either the upper or lower lip, or both lips).

Facial Plastic Surgery Network—Lip Reduction
<http://www.facialplasticsurgery.net/lip_reduction.htm>

This page can be reached directly via the URL, or go to the main page <http://www.facialplasticsurgery.net>, select "Facial Procedures," and then "Lip Reduction." This page is similar (whether you are a candidate for surgery, procedure description, expectations, recovery, risks, and complications, etc.) to Yes They're Fake! (see as follows), but without the informal, chatty comments.

Yes They're Fake!—Lip Reduction
<http://www.yestheyrefake.net/lip_reduction.htm>

This site was created by a patient who has undergone cosmetic surgery herself. The page on lip reduction (see Figure 7.9) can be located directly via the URL, or go to the main page <http://www.yestheyrefake.net>, select "Facial Procedures," and then "Lip Reduction." The page helps you decide if you are a candidate for lip surgery, describes the surgery and postsurgical recovery, and lists risks and complications.

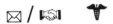

MENTOPLASTY

See CHIN AUGMENTATION (MENTOPLASTY) (in this chapter). *See also* FACIAL IMPLANTS (in this chapter).

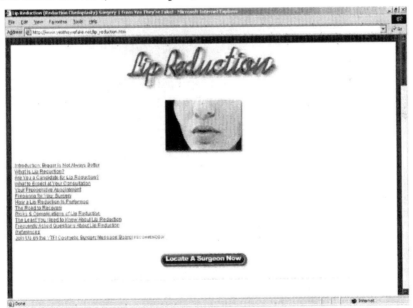

FIGURE 7.9. Yes They're Fake!—Lip Reduction
<http://www.yestheyrefake.net/lip_reduction.htm>
Reprinted with permission of Enhancement Media.

MICRODERMABRASION

See MICRODERMABRASION in Chapter 8, "Cosmetic Surgery of the Skin."

NECK LIFT/NECK LIPOSUCTION

A neck lift is surgery that reduces/removes the sagging skin of the neck or removes excess fat in the neck area, giving the jaw a more defined look and eliminating wrinkles. A neck lift is often performed in conjunction with a facelift or other facial procedures.

Facial Plastic Surgery Network—Neck Lift
<http://www.facialplasticsurgery.net/neck_lift.htm>

This page can be reached directly via the URL, or go to the main page <http://www.facialplasticsurgery.net>, select "Facial Procedures," and then "Neck Lift." This page is similar (whether you are a candidate for surgery, procedure description, expectations, recovery, risks and complications, etc.) to Yes They're Fake! (see as follows), but without the informal, chatty comments.

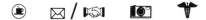

iEnhance—Neck Liposuction
<http://www.ienhance.com/procedure/default.asp>

Go directly to the "Procedures" page and select either "Plastic Surgery" or "Facial Plastic Surgery," then under "Head/Face" select "Neck Liposuction." The page includes basic information such as whether you are a candidate for surgery, surgical procedure, risks, postsurgical recovery, and questions to ask your doctor.

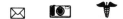

Yes They're Fake!—Neck Lift
<http://www.yestheyrefake.net/neck_lift.htm>

The page on neck lift can be located directly via the URL, or go to the main page <http://www.yestheyrefake.net>, select "Facial Procedures," and then "Neck Lift." The page describes what a neck lift is, whether you are a candidate for a neck lift, how a neck lift is performed, the recovery, risks and complications, and more.

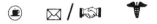

NOSE SURGERY (RHINOPLASTY)

Rhinoplasty, or surgery of the nose ("nose job"), is performed for both cosmetic purposes, or for functional reasons, i.e., to improve breathing. Reshaping of the nose—changing the size and shape—has a major impact on one's appearance, and thus it is one of the most common cosmetic procedures.

2003 statistics:

ASAPS: 172,420 (119,047 in women)
ASPS: 356,554 (226,780 in women)

American Academy of Cosmetic Surgery—Rhinoplasty (Surgery of the Nose)
<http://www.cosmeticsurgery.org/procedures/rhinoplasty.asp?mn=pc>

Go directly to the URL, or select "Patient Center," then "Learn About a Cosmetic Procedure," then "Rhinoplasty (Surgery of the Nose)." The page contains basic information about surgery of the nose, whether you are a candidate for this surgery, pre- and postsurgery information, and risks.

American Academy of Facial Plastic and Reconstructive Surgery— Understanding Rhinoplasty Surgery
<http://www.aafprs.org/patient/procedures/rhinoplasty.html>

The AAFPRS patient information includes a description of the procedure, deciding on nose surgery, postsurgery information, and before/after illustrations.

American Academy of Otolaryngology—Head and Neck Surgery— Surgery of the Nose
<http://www.entnet.org/healthinfo/nose/surgery_nose.cfm>

The AAO-HNS site discusses surgery of the nose both for cosmetic and functional reasons (e.g., nasal obstruction). Before/after illustrations are available.

American Society for Aesthetic Plastic Surgery—Nose Reshaping
<http://www.surgery.org/public/procedures-nosereshape.php>

This ASAPS public page on nose reshaping (see Figure 7.10) leads to additional pages containing information about the surgical procedure, risks, before and after surgery, and more. This is one of the better sites available about rhinoplasty.

American Society of Plastic Surgeons—Rhinoplasty (Surgery of the Nose)
<http://www.plasticsurgery.org/public_education/procedures/ Rhinoplasty.cfm>

The ASPS public information page on surgery of the nose (see Figure 7.11) includes a description of the surgery, anesthesia, risks, postsurgical recovery, and before/after illustrations. This page is available in Spanish (choose Spanish from Procedures page or go directly to <http://www. plasticsurgery.org/public_education/procedures/Rinoplastia.cfm>).

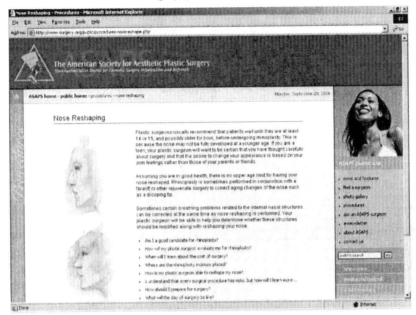

FIGURE 7.10. American Society for Aesthetic Plastic Surgery—Nose Reshaping
<http://www.surgery.org/public/procedures-nosereshape.php>
Reprinted with permission of American Society for Aesthetic Plastic Surgery.

Bermant Plastic and Cosmetic Surgery
<http://www.plasticsurgery4u.com>

This site is provided by Dr. Michael Bermant, a board certified physician in plastic surgery, who practices near Richmond, VA. Although the site is not well organized, it contains a wealth of information. Scroll until you get to "Nasal Sculpture" and then link to a wealth of information about rhinoplasty, from the procedure itself to ethnic issues. The site subscribes to the HONcode principles.

iEnhance—Nose Surgery (Rhinoplasty)
<http://www.ienhance.com/procedure/default.asp>

Go directly to the Procedure page and select either "Plastic Surgery" or "Facial Plastic Surgery," then under "Head/Face" select "Nose Surgery

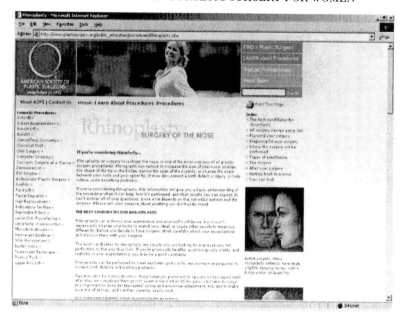

FIGURE 7.11. American Society of Plastic Surgeons—Rhinoplasty (Surgery of the Nose)
<http://www.plasticsurgery.org/public_education/procedures/Rhinoplasty.cfm>
© 2004 American Society of Plastic Surgeons. All rights reserved. Learn more at <www.plasticsurgery.org>.

(Rhinoplasty)." The page includes basic information such as patient selection, surgical procedure, risks, postsurgical recovery, and questions to ask your doctor.

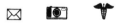

Rhinoplasty 4 You
<http://www.rhinoplasty4you.com>

This site is produced by Enhancement Media and is part of the Facial Plastic Surgery network sites <http://www.facialplasticsurgery.net>. It is easy to navigate with links on the left-hand side for "Understanding the Nose," "Researching the Procedure" (includes a glossary, surgical procedure details, risks, and complications), "Road to Recovery," and a photo gallery (linked under "Miscellaneous Information"), and more. Visit also All About Revision Rhinoplasty <http://www.revisionrhinoplasty.net>. Included in "Surgeon Information" are tips on how to choose a good surgeon and how to research the surgeon's credentials.

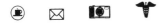

Rhinoplasty FYI
<http://www.rhinoplastyfyi.com>

A special section of the Cosmetic Surgery FYI site, this site gives extensive information about the rhinoplasty surgical procedure and patient expectations, who is a candidate for surgery, and risks. It contains links to before/after photos. There is a link to the surgeon locator on each page, plus financing information.

Yes They're Fake!—Rhinoplasty
<http://www.yestheyrefake.net/rhinoplasty.html>

This is a refreshingly candid site, created by a patient who has undergone cosmetic surgery herself. The page on Rhinoplasty (nose surgery) can be located directly via the URL, or go to the main page <http://www.yestheyrefake.net>, select "Facial Procedures," and then "Rhinoplasty." The page discusses whether you are a candidate for rhinoplasty, risks and complications, and depression after rhinoplasty; also included are FAQs about rhinoplasty, a before-and-after photo gallery, and a rhinoplasty message board. Also check out the links to "Revision Rhinoplasty" <http://www.yestheyrefake.net/revision_rhinoplasty.thm> and "Septoplasty" <http://www.yestheyrefake.net/septoplasty.htm>. A link refers you to Rhinoplasty 4 You <http://www.rhinoplasty.com> (see earlier listing).

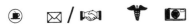

OTOPLASTY

See EAR SURGERY (in this chapter).

RHINOPLASTY

See NOSE SURGERY (in this chapter).

RHYTIDECTOMY

See FACELIFT (in this chapter).

Chapter 8

Cosmetic Surgery of the Skin

This chapter reviews cosmetic procedures of the skin, covering all parts of the body, including the face. The majority of cosmetic surgery procedures for the skin are designed to combat the aging process, e.g., wrinkles, sagging skin, rough/irregular patches of skin. However, some procedures such as tattoo removal or scar revision are cosmetic in nature, but are not related to aging.

Procedures in this chapter include nonsurgical treatments, laser treatments, resurfacing, and injections. Because so many of these procedures have multiple uses, and many of the conditions have options for treatment, it was difficult to organize this chapter. You are encouraged to browse this entire chapter rather than focus on a specific procedure, as many sites offer different approaches to a topic. Cross-references will direct you to appropriate sections in this chapter or to other chapters.

Surgical procedures intended to reshape the face, head, and neck are covered in Chapter 7, "Cosmetic Surgery of the Face, Head, and Neck." Hair replacement is covered in Chapter 9, "Hair Transplantation for Women." If you are unable to locate a procedure, please check the Index.

SKIN—GENERAL

AgingSkinNet
<http://www.skincarephysicians.com/agingskinnet/index.html>

AgingSkinNet is "an educational program brought to you by the American Academy of Dermatology." Within this site is a section, "Cosmetic Procedures," which provides brief information about a variety of procedures, both surgical and nonsurgical, that can be used to treat aging skin. Other pages include information on hair loss and choosing a dermatologist.

American Academy of Dermatology—Public Resource Center— Pamphlets
<http://www.aad.org/public/Publications/PamphletsIntro.htm>

For patient information from the American Academy of Dermatology, it's best to go directly to the URL (see Figure 8.1). However, if you choose to begin at the home page <http://www.aad.org>, select "Public Resource Center" and then, from the lower left-hand side of the page, "Publications," followed by "Pamphlets." Pamphlets range from cosmetic surgery topics to dermatologic conditions. "Press Releases" (select "News & Events," then "Press Releases") also has useful information for patients.

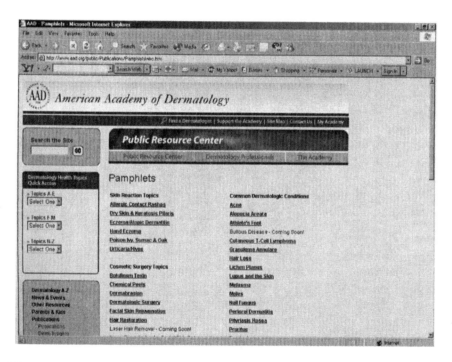

FIGURE 8.1. American Academy of Dermatology—Public Resource Center— Pamphlets
<http://www.aad.org/public/Publications/PamphletsIntro.htm>
© 2004 American Academy of Dermatology. Used with permission.

American Society for Dermatologic Surgery
<http://www.asds.net/Patients/patients-procedures.html>

The American Society for Dermatologic Surgery (ASDS) is a membership organization of board certified dermatologic surgeons. The ASDS site offers information both for patients and members of the society. The "Dermatologic Surgical Procedures" page (see Figure 8.2) links to fact sheets on procedures and techniques, definitions, and photographs. Procedures include treatment/surgery for skin conditions such as acne scars, skin cancer, and tattoo removal, but also procedures such as hair restoration, liposuction, and eyelid surgery. Selecting "Your Skin Surgery Expert" connects you to information about training and services provided by dermatologic surgeons, along with summary information on procedures and photographs. "Find a Dermatologic Surgeon" helps locate a surgeon

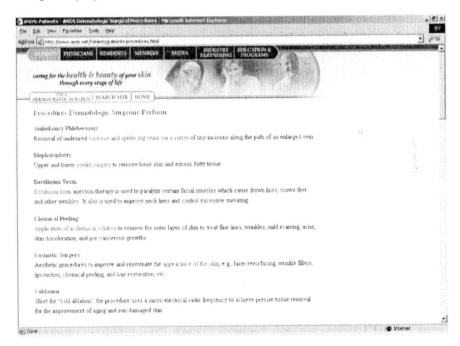

FIGURE 8.2. American Society for Dermatologic Surgery—Dermatologic Surgical Procedures
<http://www.asds.net/Patients/patients-procedures.html>
Reprinted with permission of American Society for Dermatologic Surgery.

near you; also accessible are member pages with contact information and procedures performed.

Facial Plastic Surgery Network
<http://www.facialplasticsurgery.net>

"The Facial Plastic Surgery Network is dedicated to helping you obtain solutions to your facial aesthetic concerns." This site is produced by Enhancement Media, a company that has a group of "sister" sites on many cosmetic surgery topics. The site is easy to navigate, with links at the top of the home page to pages on "Facial Procedures," "Choosing a Surgeon," "Procedure FAQ," "Anesthesia Information," a photo gallery, chat groups and discussion forums, and more. A key page is "Facial Procedures" (see Figure 7.2 in Chapter 7), which has links to an extensive list of procedures (some of these are individually listed later in this chapter and also in Chapter 7, "Cosmetic Surgery of the Face, Head, and Neck"). About half of the procedures listed on this page are skin related. Information is similar to the site Yes They're Fake! which is also produced by the same company.

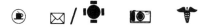

iEnhance—Facial Plastic Surgery
<http://www.ienhance.com/speciality/facial.asp>

Cosmetic procedures of the skin are included by iEnhance in their "Facial Plastic Surgery" page. Go directly to the URL (*sic*—speciality in URL), or begin at the general <http://www.ienhance.com> and select "Facial Plastic Surgery." This page has links to featured articles, archived articles, a photo gallery, a doctor locator, and specific surgical procedures. Select "Procedures" from this page, and then "Facial Plastic Surgery" to link to information on twenty-five to thirty facial plastic surgery procedures (see Figure 7.3 in Chapter 7), from dermabrasion and chemical peel to laser hair removal and Botox. Included are surgical procedures of the face (see Chapter 7) and hair transplantation (see Chapter 9).

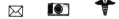

Yes They're Fake!—Facial Enhancement
<http://www.yestheyrefake.net/facial_plastic_surgery.html>

This is a refreshingly candid site, created by a patient who has undergone cosmetic surgery herself. Go directly to the URL, or go to the main page <http://www.yestheyrefake.net>, and select "Facial Procedures." A majority of the specific procedures from the "Facial Enhancement" page (see Figure 7.4 in Chapter 7) are listed later in this chapter (or in Chapter 7, "Cosmetic Surgery of the Face, Head, and Neck") under the specific procedure, but it was not possible to list all (e.g., "Hyperpigmentation Removal," "Intense Pulsed Light," and "Thermage [Thermacool TC]"). For those that object to the informality of this site, go to Facial Plastic Surgery Network <http://www.facialplasticsurgery.net> for similar information without the personal commentary.

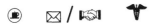

BOTULINUM TOXIN (BOTOX) INJECTIONS

Botulinum toxin (Botox) is a toxin that is injected into the skin to remove wrinkles and lines. Originally used to treat neurological disorders, Botox works by blocking nerve impulses, thus paralyzing muscles that can cause wrinkles. Botox is frequently injected into the forehead and lower face to reduce lines and wrinkles, and around the eyes to eliminate "crow's-feet." Botox is one of the most popular nonsurgical cosmetic procedures available today. News reports and stories abound about "Botox parties," where people gather for injections. Be sure that the person administering Botox is a board certified physician trained in this procedure.

2003 statistics:
ASAPS: 2,272,080 (1,963,012 in women)
ASPS: 2,891,390 (2,557,834 in women)

American Academy of Dermatology—Botulinum Toxin
<http://www.aad.org/public/Publications/pamphlets/Botulinum
Toxin.htm>

This AAD pamphlet describes botulinum toxin (Botox), use of Botox for wrinkles, how it works, and side effects.

American Academy of Facial Plastic and Reconstructive Surgery— Botox Injections
<http://www.aafprs.org/media/media_resources/fact_botox.html>

AAFPRS provides brief information about Botox injections. The site cautions that Botox injections are a medical procedure which should be performed by a qualified facial plastic surgeon under appropriate conditions using sterile techniques.

American Society for Aesthetic Plastic Surgery—Botulinum Toxin Injections
<http://www.surgery.org/public/procedures-botoxing.php>

This ASAPS public page on Botox injections describes uses for botulinum toxin, the technique, benefits, and other considerations, along with an ASAPS position statement on the procedure.

American Society for Dermatologic Surgery—Botulinum Toxin Treatments
<http://www.asds.net/Patients/FactSheets/patients-Fact_Sheet-botulinum_toxin.html>

Go directly to the URL or select "Patients," then "Fact Sheets," and then "Botulinum Toxin Treatments." This ASDS fact sheet about Botox includes information about the toxin, how and where it is used, what to expect after treatment, and side effects.

American Society of Plastic Surgeons—Facial Rejuvenation (Botox)
<http://www.plasticsurgery.org/public_education/procedures/Botox.cfm>

The ASPS page on Botox provides a brief description about the injections and what the toxin does, but lists no side effects.

iEnhance—Botox Injections
<http://www.ienhance.com/procedure/default.asp>

Go directly to the "Procedures" page and select either "Plastic Surgery" or "Facial Plastic Surgery," then under "Head/Face" select "Botox Injections." The page includes basic information on the procedure, its benefits, risks, outcome, the ideal candidate for the procedure, and questions to ask your doctor.

MedlinePlus—Botox
<http://www.nlm.nih.gov/medlineplus/botox.html>

The "Botox" page on MedlinePlus (see Figure 8.3) directs you to quality information on Botox, including government and association sites. It's a good place to start.

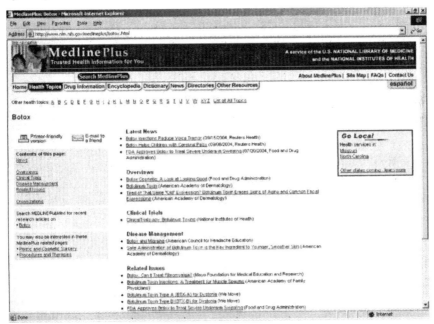

FIGURE 8.3. MedlinePlus—Botox
<http://www.nlm.nih.gov/medlineplus/botox.html>

U.S. Food and Drug Administration—Botox Cosmetic: A Look at Looking Good
<http://www.fda.gov/fdac/features/2002/402_botox.html>

This is an article, "Botox Cosmetic: A Look at Looking Good," that was published in the July-August 2002 *FDA Consumer* magazine (see Figure 8.4). It explains how Botox works, mentions Botox "parties" and includes an FDA recommendation on use. Also available from the FDA is a Botox fact sheet at <http://www.fda.gov/womens/getthefacts/botox.html>.

Yes They're Fake!—Botox
<http://www.yestheyrefake.net/botox.htm>

This is a refreshingly candid site, created by a patient who has undergone cosmetic surgery herself. Go directly to the URL, or go to the main

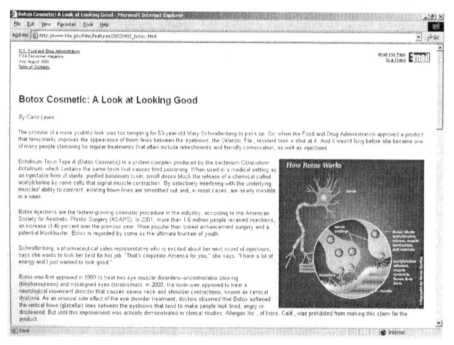

FIGURE 8.4. U.S. FDA—Botox Cosmetic
<http://www.fda.gov/fdac/features/2002/402_botox.html>

page <http://www.yestheyrefake.net>, select "Facial Procedures," and then "Botox." The page discusses what Botox is and what it's used for, where it can be injected, what to expect, and risks, complications, and contraindications.

CELLULITE TREATMENT

Cellulite is the "dimplelike" fat that occurs in women, frequently in the thighs, abdomen, and buttock areas. Treatments range from creams to liposuction, with varying levels of success.

2003 statistics:

ASAPS:	27,919	(26,558 in women)
ASPS:	44,579	(38,655 in women)

American Academy of Dermatology—Dermatologists Shed Light on Treatments for Cellulite
<http://www.aad.org>

At the AAD site, do a site search for "cellulite" to find this archived press release, which describes cellulite and its treatments—creams, mechanical massage, diet, and exercise. According to the AAD, there is no permanent solution.

American Skincare and Cellulite Expert Association
<http://www.ascea.org>

According to the Web site, "ASCEA is the largest and most innovative professional association serving the needs of hundreds of cellulite treatment centers in 20-plus countries." This site has information on cellulite anatomy (showing how women store fat differently than men), treatments, Endermologie (a trademarked system for "subdermal treatment for reducing cellulite"), and a directory of accredited centers.

WebMD—Getting Rid of Cellulite
<http://www.webmd.com>

Go to the general WebMD page, and search for "cellulite." One result is a featured article from the archive, "Getting Rid of Cellulite," which discusses what cellulite is and various treatments available, mostly over the counter. Most treatment options are considered ineffective.

Yes They're Fake!—Cellulite Treatment
<http://www.yestheyrefake.net/cellulite_treatment_removal.htm>

Go directly to the URL, or go to the main page <http://www.yestheyrefake.net>, select "Body Procedures," and then "Cellulite Treatment." The page reviews what cellulite is versus "normal" fat, treatment options (from Endermologie to liposuction to RejuveSkin), and discusses whether you are a candidate for cellulite removal, plus complications and risks. Also, check out another page on this site dedicated to "RejuveSkin Treatment for Cellulite" <http://www.yestheyrefake.net/rejuveskin_cellulite.htm>. (Another page on Endermologie was incomplete at the time of this review.)

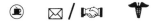

CHEMICAL PEELS

Chemical peels involve using a chemical solution on the surface of the skin to peel away the top layers of the skin. Factors such as the strength of the chemical and how long it is left on the skin will determine how many layers of skin are peeled away. Chemical peels are used to treat skin conditions such as wrinkles and imperfections in the skin (e.g., acne scars). Skin that is regenerated after chemical peeling is smoother and has less wrinkles than before. Chemical peels can be used with other procedures such as dermabrasion; this procedure is not a substitute for a facelift.

2003 statistics:

ASAPS:	722,248	(640,081 in women)
ASPS:	995,238	(891,321 in women)

American Academy of Cosmetic Surgery—Chemical Peels
<http://www.cosmeticsurgery.org/procedures/chemical_peels.asp? mn=pc>

Go directly to the URL, or select "Patient Center," then "Learn About a Cosmetic Procedure," then "Chemical Peels." Contains basic information about the procedure, pre- and postsurgery information, and risks.

American Academy of Dermatology—Chemical Peeling
<http://www.aad.org/public/Publications/pamphlets/chempeel.htm>

This AAD pamphlet describes what chemical peeling can do, how it is performed, what to expect after treatment, possible complications, and limitations of the procedure.

American Society for Aesthetic Plastic Surgery—Chemical Skin Peel (Light and Deep)
<http://www.surgery.org/public/procedures-chem_peel_light.php>
<http://www.surgery.org/public/procedures-chem_peel_deep.php>

The ASAPS has two public pages on chemical skin peels: one discusses light to medium peels, the second reviews deep (phenol) peels. Each page describes uses for chemical peels, the technique, benefits, and other considerations. The deep-peel page indicates what to expect after the procedure.

American Society for Dermatologic Surgery—Chemical Peeling
<http://www.asds.net/Patients/FactSheets/patients-Fact_Sheet-chem_peel.html>

Go directly to the URL, or select "Patients," then "Fact Sheets," and then "Chemical Peeling." This ASDS fact sheet about chemical peeling includes information about the procedure, why it's performed, and what to expect after treatment.

American Society of Plastic Surgeons—Chemical Peel
<http://www.plasticsurgery.org/public_education/procedures/chemicalpeel.cfm>

The ASPS page on chemical peels (see Figure 8.5) provides fairly extensive information, including a general overview, preparing for a chemical peel, the procedure itself, and posttreatment. Three chemical solutions are described along with specific uses and considerations for each formula. Includes illustrations.

Facial Plastic Surgery Network—Chemical Peels
<http://www.facialplasticsurgery.net/chemical_peel.htm>

This page can be reached directly via the URL, or go to the main page <http://www.facialplasticsurgery.net>, select "Facial Procedures," and then "Chemical Peel." This page is similar (whether you are a candidate for the procedure, procedure description with options, expectations, recovery, risks, and complications) to Yes They're Fake! (see as follows), but without the informal, chatty comments.

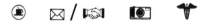

iEnhance—Chemical Peel
<http://www.ienhance.com/procedure/default.asp>

Go directly to the "Procedures" page and select either "Plastic Surgery" or "Facial Plastic Surgery," then under "Head/Face" select "Chemical Peel." Includes basic information such as surgical procedure, risks, postsurgical recovery, the ideal candidate for the procedure, and questions to ask your doctor.

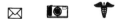

Yes They're Fake!—Chemical Peels
<http://www.yestheyrefake.net/chemical_peel.htm>

This is a refreshingly candid site, created by a patient who has undergone cosmetic surgery herself. Go directly to the URL, or go to the main

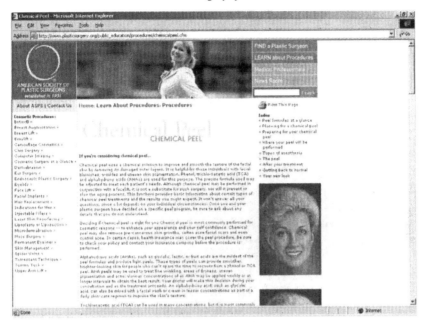

FIGURE 8.5. American Society of Plastic Surgeons—Chemical Peel
<http://www.plasticsurgery.org/public_education/procedures/chemicalpeel.cfm>

page <http://www.yestheyrefake.net>, select "Facial Procedures," and then "Chemical Peels." The page covers options for chemical peels, preoperative information, how the procedure is performed, the recovery, contraindications, and risks and complications.

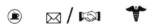

COLLAGEN INJECTIONS

See under INJECTABLE FILLERS (in this chapter).

DERMABRASION

Dermabrasion is used to treat facial skin conditions such as acne scars, wrinkles, sun damage, and scars from accidents. The patient's skin is numbed and then the surgeon scrapes, or planes, the outer layer of skin. The new skin that forms under the treated area has a smoother appearance.

2003 statistics:

ASAPS: 27,584 (22,775 in women)
ASPS: 60,255 (51,488 in women)

American Academy of Cosmetic Surgery—Laser Surfacing and Dermabrasion
<http://www.cosmeticsurgery.org/procedures/laser_surfacing_and_ dermabrasi.asp?mn=pc>

Go directly to the URL, or select "Patient Center," then "Learn About a Cosmetic Procedure," then "Laser Resurfacing and Dermabrasion." The page contains basic information about each procedure, whether you are a good candidate, pre- and postsurgery information, and risks. For costs, you are referred to your cosmetic surgeon.

American Academy of Dermatology—Dermabrasion
<http://www.aad.org/public/Publications/pamphlets/dermabrasion. htm>

This AAD pamphlet describes dermabrasion, indications for the procedure, how it is performed, possible complications, and limitations of the procedure.

American Society for Dermatologic Surgery—Dermabrasion
<http://www.asds.net/Patients/FactSheets/patients-Fact_Sheet- dermabrasion.html>

Go directly to the URL, or select "Patients," then "Fact Sheets," and then "Dermabrasion." This ASDS fact sheet about chemical peeling describes the procedure, when it should be used, and what to expect before, during, and after treatment.

American Society of Plastic Surgeons—Dermabrasion
<http://www.plasticsurgery.org/public_education/procedures/ dermabrasion.cfm>

The ASPS page on dermabrasion (see Figure 8.6) provides fairly extensive information, including a general overview, alternative procedures, best candidates for the treatment, risks, preparing for dermabrasion, the surgery itself, and posttreatment.

Facial Plastic Surgery Network—Dermabrasion
<http://www.facialplasticsurgery.net/dermabrasion.htm>

This page can be reached directly via the URL, or go to the main page <http://www.facialplasticsurgery.net>, select "Facial Procedures," and then "Dermabrasion." This page is similar (whether you are a candidate for the procedure, procedure description, expectations, recovery, risks, and complications) to Yes They're Fake!

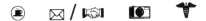

iEnhance—Dermabrasion
<http://www.ienhance.com/procedure/default.asp>

Go directly to the "Procedures" page and select either "Plastic Surgery" or "Facial Plastic Surgery," then under "Head/Face" select "Dermabrasion." The page includes basic information on the procedure, risks, postsurgical recovery, the ideal candidate for the procedure, and questions to ask your doctor.

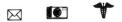

Yes They're Fake!—Dermabrasion
<http://www.yestheyrefake.net/dermabrasion.htm>

This is a refreshingly candid site, created by a patient who has undergone cosmetic surgery herself. Go directly to the URL, or go to the main page <http://www.yestheyrefake.net>, select "Facial Procedures," and then "Dermabrasion." The page covers whether you are a candidate for

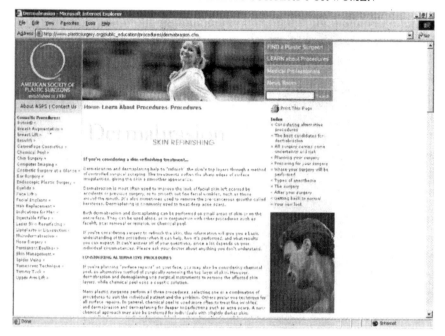

FIGURE 8.6. American Society of Plastic Surgeons—Dermabrasion
<http://www.plasticsurgery.org/public_education/procedures/dermabrasion.cfm>
© 2004 American Society of Plastic Surgeons. All rights reserved. Learn more at
    <www.plasticsurgery.org>.

dermabrasion, preoperative information, how the procedure is performed, the recovery, and risks and complications.

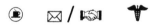

ENDERMOLOGIE

See CELLULITE TREATMENT (in this chapter).

FAT INJECTIONS

See under INJECTABLE FILLERS (in this chapter).

HAIR REPLACEMENT

See Chapter 9, "Hair Transplantation for Women."

INJECTABLE FILLERS

Injectable fillers are another form of cosmetic treatment used to make acne scars, wrinkles, and other facial skin imperfections less noticeable, and to restore a more youthful appearance to the skin. The most commonly used fillers are collagen and fat (each will be discussed in later sections). These fillers, when injected under the skin, eliminate wrinkles and make the skin look smoother. This treatment can be combined with other cosmetic procedures, such as facial resurfacing or a facelift.

American Academy of Dermatology—Soft Tissue Fillers
<http://www.aad.org/public/Publications/pamphlets/
SoftTissueFillers.htm>

This AAD page reviews soft tissue fillers and what they can do; briefly describes several types of fillers, and describes the procedure, risks, and treatment options.

American Society of Plastic Surgeons—Injectable Fillers
<http://www.plasticsurgery.org/public_education/procedures/
injectablefillers.cfm>

This ASPS page discusses what fillers are used for, options to fillers, risks, and the procedure (with a focus on collagen and fat fillers).

Facial Plastic Surgery Network—Injectables: Fillers for Soft Tissue
Augmentation
<http://www.facialplasticsurgery.net/injectable_fillers.htm>

This page can be reached directly via the URL, or go to the main page <http://www.facialplasticsurgery.net>, select "Facial Procedures," and then "Injectable Fillers." This page links to five pages of augmentation materials, by category: "Temporary Injectables," "Permanent Injectable Micro-implants," "Injectable Bio-catalysts," "Injectable Bio-implants," and "Injectable Self-derivative Products."

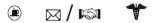

iEnhance—Skin Injection Treatments
<http://www.ienhance.com/procedure/default.asp>

Go directly to the "Procedures" page and select either "Plastic Surgery" or "Facial Plastic Surgery," then under "Head/Face" select "Skin Injection Treatments." The page includes benefits of the procedure, risks, postsurgical recovery, the ideal candidate for the procedure, and questions to ask your doctor. Injectables mentioned are: AlloDerm (including Cymetra), Botox, collagen, fat, and silicone.

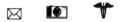

Collagen Injections

2003 statistics:

ASAPS:	620,476	(568,797 in women)
ASPS:	576,255	(547,874 in women)

American Society for Aesthetic Plastic Surgery—Collagen Injections
<http://www.surgery.org/public/procedures-collagen.php>

This ASAPS public page on collagen injections describes uses for collagen injections, the technique, benefits, and other considerations.

Fat Injections

2003 statistics:

ASAPS:	90,321	(83,295 in women)
ASPS:	61,852	(55,591 in women)

American Society for Aesthetic Plastic Surgery—Fat Injection
<http://www.surgery.org/public/procedures-fatinject.php>

This ASAPS public page on fat injection describes uses for fat injections, the technique, benefits, and other considerations. In the "Photo Gallery," look under "Soft Tissue Fillers."

American Society for Dermatologic Surgery—Microlipoinjection (or Fat Transfer)
<http://www.asds.net/Patients/FactSheets/patients-Fact_Sheet-microlipoinjection.html>

Go directly to the URL, or select "Patients," then "Fact Sheets," and then "Microlipoinjection." This ASDS fact sheet about microlipoinjection describes the procedure and its uses.

Facial Plastic Surgery Network—Facial Fat Grafting (Fat Transfer)
<http://www.facialplasticsurgery.net/fat_grafting.htm>

This page can be reached directly via the URL, or go to the main page <http://www.facialplasticsurgery.net>, select "Facial Procedures," and then "Fat Grafting." This page is similar (whether you are a candidate for the procedure, procedure description, expectations, recovery, risks and complications, and more) to Yes They're Fake! (see as follows), but without the informal, chatty comments.

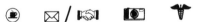

iEnhance—Fat Injections
<http://www.ienhance.com/procedure/default.asp>

Go directly to the "Procedures" page and select either "Plastic Surgery" or "Facial Plastic Surgery," then under "Head/Face" select "Fat Injections." The page includes basic information about the surgical procedure, benefits, risks, postsurgical recovery, the ideal candidate for the procedure, and questions to ask your doctor.

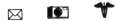

Yes They're Fake!—Fat Grafting
<http://www.yestheyrefake.net/fat_grafting.htm>

This is a refreshingly candid site, created by a patient who has undergone cosmetic surgery herself. Go directly to the URL, or go to the main page <http://www.yestheyrefake.net>, select "Facial Procedures," and then "Fat Grafting/Transfer." The page describes the procedure, whether you are a good candidate, expectations, the recovery, and risks and complications.

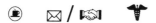

LASER HAIR REMOVAL

Laser hair removal is a popular, new treatment for permanent removal of unwanted hair from the face or body. A low-energy laser is applied through the skin into the hair follicle, thus damaging the follicle and stopping hair growth.

2003 statistics:

ASAPS:	923,200	(695,210 in women)
ASPS:	623,297	(450,018 in women)

American Society for Aesthetic Plastic Surgery—Laser Hair Removal
<http://www.surgery.org/public/procedures-hairremove.php>

This ASAPS public page on hair removal contains information about this nonsurgical procedure, benefits, and other considerations. Laser hair removal is used on the face and other parts of the body.

American Society for Dermatologic Surgery—Laser Hair Removal
<http://www.asds.net/Patients/FactSheets/patients-Fact_Sheet-laser_hair_removal.html>

Go directly to the URL, or select "Patients," then "Fact Sheets," and then "Laser Hair Removal." This ASDS fact sheet about laser hair removal includes information about hair growth, the laser hair removal procedure, types of lasers, and the advantages and limitations of laser hair removal.

iEnhance—Laser Hair Removal
<http://www.ienhance.com/procedure/default.asp>

Go directly to the "Procedures" page and select either "Plastic Surgery" or "Facial Plastic Surgery," then under "Head/Face" select "Laser Hair Removal." The page includes basic information on the procedure, risks, what to expect afterward, the ideal candidate for the procedure, and questions to ask your doctor.

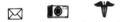

MayoClinic.com—Laser Hair Removal: Zapping Unwanted Hair
<http://www.mayoclinic.com/invoke.cfm?id=HQ00981>

Go directly to the URL, or go to the general Mayo site <http://www. mayoclinic.com> and do a site search for "laser hair removal." This page describes the procedure along with advantages and disadvantages over other procedures.

LASER SKIN RESURFACING

Laser skin resurfacing is used to remove wrinkles, scars, and areas of damaged skin. It can be used on the whole face, but is especially helpful in minimizing lines around the eyes ("crow's-feet") and mouth. Lasers can be more precise than chemical peels or dermabrasion. Laser resurfacing is often done in combination with another procedure such as eyelid surgery or a facelift.

2003 statistics:

ASAPS:	127,470	(116,467 in women)
ASPS:	180,855	(167,662 in women)

American Academy of Cosmetic Surgery—Laser Surfacing and Dermabrasion
<http://www.cosmeticsurgery.org/procedures/laser_surfacing_and_ dermabrasi.asp?mn=pc>

Go directly to the URL, or select "Patient Center," then "Learn About a Cosmetic Procedure," then "Laser Resurfacing and Dermabrasion." This page contains basic information about each procedure, whether you are a good candidate, pre- and postsurgery information, and risks. For costs, you are referred to your cosmetic surgeon.

American Academy of Dermatology—Laser Resurfacing for Facial Skin Rejuvenation
<http://www.aad.org/public/Publications/pamphlets/ LaserResurfacingRejuv.htm>

This AAD pamphlet describes the procedure of laser resurfacing, types of lasers and what they are used for, what to expect during and after the treatment, and possible complications and limitations of the procedure.

American Society for Dermatologic Surgery—Laser Resurfacing
<http://www.asds.net/Patients/FactSheets/patients-Fact_Sheet-laser_resurfacing.html>

Go directly to the URL, or select "Patients," then "Fact Sheets," and then "Laser Resurfacing." This ASDS fact sheet about laser resurfacing describes the procedure, why it's performed, types of lasers (more can be found under "Laser Applications"), what to expect during and after treatment, and side effects/complications.

American Society of Plastic Surgeons—Laser Skin Resurfacing
<http://www.plasticsurgery.org/public_education/procedures/Laser-Skin-Resurfacing.cfm>

This ASPS page on laser skin resurfacing provides a brief description about the procedure and what it is used for, but lists no side effects. More extensive information is available from the "Reconstructive Procedures" list that includes skin resurfacing <http://www.plasticsurgery.org/public_education/procedures/SkinResurfacing.cfm>.

Facial Plastic Surgery Network—Laser Resurfacing & Laser Treatments
<http://www.facialplasticsurgery.net/laser_resurfacing.htm>

This page can be reached directly via the URL, or go to the main page <http://www.facialplasticsurgery.net>, select "Facial Procedures," and then "LASER Resurfacing." This page is similar to Yes They're Fake! (see as follows), but without the informal, chatty comments. The page describes lasers and how they work, laser resurfacing and types of lasers, plus how laser resurfacing is performed and whether you are a candidate, the recovery, and risks and complications. Also check out the page on "NLite Laser" <http://www.facialplasticsurgery.net/NLite.htm>.

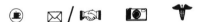

iEnhance—Laser Skin Resurfacing
<http://www.ienhance.com/procedure/default.asp>

Go directly to the "Procedures" page and select either "Plastic Surgery" or "Facial Plastic Surgery," then under "Head/Face" select "Laser Skin Resurfacing." The page includes basic information such as surgical procedure, types of lasers, risks, postsurgical recovery, the ideal candidate for the procedure, and questions to ask your doctor.

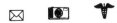

MayoClinic.com—Laser Resurfacing: One Way to Treat Wrinkles
\<http://www.mayoclinic.com/invoke.cfm?id=WO00008\>

Go directly to the URL, or go to the general Mayo site \<http://www. mayoclinic.com\> and do a site search for "laser resurfacing" or "wrinkles." The procedure is described along with what to expect from the surgery, recovery information, complications and risks, and the need for realistic expectations for the surgery.

Yes They're Fake!—Laser Treatments
\<http://www.yestheyrefake.net/laser_resurfacing.htm\>

This is a refreshingly candid site, created by a patient who has undergone cosmetic surgery herself. Go directly to the URL, or go to the main page \<http://www.yestheyrefake.net\>, select "Facial Procedures," and then "Laser Treatments." The page describes lasers and how they work, laser resurfacing and types of lasers, plus how laser resurfacing is performed and whether you are a candidate, the recovery, and risks and complications. Also check out the page on "NLite Laser" \<http://yestheyrefake. net/NLite.htm\>.

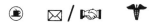

LASER TREATMENT OF SPIDER VEINS

This procedure removes spider veins using a laser. It is most frequently performed on spider veins of the face, as spider veins elsewhere on the body are normally removed with sclerotherapy.

2003 statistics:

ASAPS:	170,358	(163,149 in women)
ASPS:	113,852	(108,374 in women)

iEnhance—Laser Spider Vein Treatment
\<http://www.ienhance.com/procedure/default.asp\>

Go directly to the "Procedures" page and select either "Plastic Surgery" or "Facial Plastic Surgery," then under "Head/Face" or "Legs" select "Laser Spider Vein Treatment." The page includes basic information such as surgical procedure, risks, postsurgical recovery, the ideal candidate for the procedure, and questions to ask your doctor.

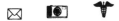

MICRODERMABRASION

Microdermabrasion is a nonsurgical treatment for fine lines and wrinkles in the face. The technique involves gentle "brushing" of the face with crystals, which stimulates production of collagen and skin cells, resulting in a more youthful appearance.

2003 statistics:

ASAPS:	858,312	(774,261 in women)
ASPS:	935,984	(694,100 in women)

**American Society for Aesthetic Plastic Surgery—
Microdermabrasion
<http://www.surgery.org/public/procedures-microderm.php>**

This ASAPS public page on microdermabrasion, a nonsurgical cosmetic procedure, contains general information about the procedure, a description of the technique, benefits, and other considerations.

**American Society of Plastic Surgeons—Microdermabrasion
<http://www.plasticsurgery.org/public_education/procedures/
Microdermabrasion.cfm>**

This ASPS page on microdermabrasion provides a brief description about microdermabrasion and what the procedure is used for, but lists no side effects.

Facial Plastic Surgery Network—Microdermabrasion
<http://www.facialplasticsurgery.net/microdermabrasion.htm>

This page (see Figure 8.7) can be reached directly via the URL, or go to the main page <http://www.facialplasticsurgery.net>, select "Facial Procedures," and then "Microdermabrasion." This page is similar (whether you are a candidate for the procedure, procedure description, expectations, recovery, risks and complications, and more) to Yes They're Fake! (see as follows).

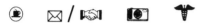

Yes They're Fake!—Microdermabrasion
<http://www.yestheyrefake.net/microdermabrasion.htm>

This is a refreshingly candid site, created by a patient who has undergone cosmetic surgery herself. Go directly to the URL, or go to the main page <http://www.yestheyrefake.net>, select "Facial Procedures," and then "Microdermabrasion." The page covers everything from whether you are a candidate for this procedure and what to expect during and after the treatment, to expectations about the procedure and risks. Included is a discussion of machines used for microdermabrasion.

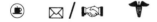

MICROPIGMENTATION (PERMANENT MAKEUP)

Micropigmentation has been given a number of names: cosmetic tattooing, dermapigmentation, and permanent makeup. For people who have allergies to cosmetics, who have difficulty putting on makeup, or who want a permanent cosmetic enhancement, this procedure has rapidly gained popularity.

American Academy of Dermatology—Tattoos, Body Piercings, and Other Skin Adornments
<http://www.aad.org/public/Publications/PamphletsIntro.htm>

The AAD Pamphlets page lists "Tattoos, Body Piercings, and Other Skin Adornments" as "Coming Soon!" Assuming the information is as

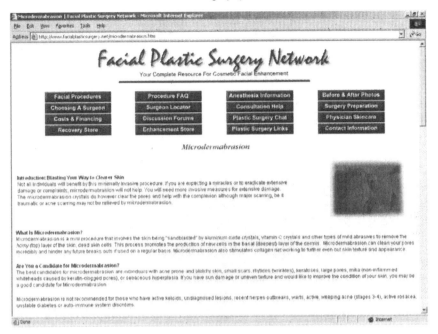

FIGURE 8.7. Facial Plastic Surgery Network—Microdermabrasion
<http://www.facialplasticsurgery.net/microdermabrasion.htm>
Reprinted with permission of Enhancement Media.

good as the other AAD public pamphlets, it is recommended. Check the
URL to link to the page.

American Society for Aesthetic Plastic Surgery—
Micropigmentation
<http://www.surgery.org/public/procedures-micropigment.php>

This ASAPS public page on micropigmentation contains general information about the procedure, benefits, and other considerations.

American Society of Plastic Surgeons—Permanent Eyeliner
<http://www.plasticsurgery.org/public_education/procedures/
Permanent-Eyeliner.cfm>

This ASPS page on permanent eyeliner is a brief description about micropigmentation, the procedure used to create permanent makeup. Benefits, but no side effects, are listed.

Facial Plastic Surgery Network—Micropigmentation (Permanent
Make Up)
<http://www.facialplasticsurgery.net/micropigmentation.htm>

This page can be reached directly via the URL, or go to the main page <http://www.facialplasticsurgery.net>, select "Facial Procedures," and then "Micropigmentation." This page is similar (what is micropigmentation, procedure description and body locations where it is done, checking the technician's background, expectations, recovery, risks and complications, and more) to Yes They're Fake!

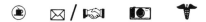

iEnhance—Permanent Cosmetics
<http://www.ienhance.com/procedure/default.asp>

Go directly to the "Procedures" page and select either "Plastic Surgery" or "Facial Plastic Surgery," then under "Head/Face" select "Permanent Cosmetics." The page includes basic information such as surgical procedure, risks, postsurgical recovery, the ideal candidate for the procedure, and questions to ask your doctor.

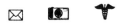

Medem—Micropigmentation (Cosmetic Tattooing)
<http://www.medem.com>

Search "Micropigmentation" in the Medem search feature to find the ASPS Briefing Paper on Micropigmentation (Cosmetic Tattooing). Provided by the American Society of Plastic Surgeons, this paper talks about the procedure, regulations, risks/complications, and recovery. This page could not be found on the ASPS page itself.

Yes They're Fake!—Micropigmentation
<http://www.yestheyrefake.net/micropigmentation.html>

This is a refreshingly candid site, created by a patient who has undergone cosmetic surgery herself. The page on micropigmentation can be located directly via the URL, or go to the main page <http://www.yestheyrefake.net>, select "Facial Procedures," and then "Micropigmentation." The page talks about what dermagraphics is, training and certifications for technicians, how the procedure is done, and areas where it is done. It is made clear that micropigmentation is tattooing.

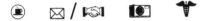

PERMANENT COSMETICS

See MICROPIGMENTATION (in this chapter).

SCARS/SCAR REVISION

Scars can be caused by accidents, burns, or surgery. With scar revision, a variety of treatments or surgery can be used to remove, relocate, or make a scar less visible.

2003 statistics:
ASPS: 232,114   (no gender breakdown)

American Academy of Dermatology—What is a Scar
<http://www.aad.org/public/Publications/pamphlets/WhatisaScar. htm>

This AAD pamphlet describes what can be done for scars; treatments range from surgical scar revision and dermabrasion to laser resurfacing and chemical peels; an extensive list of other possible treatments is given.

American Academy of Facial Plastic and Reconstructive Surgery—Understanding Facial Scar Treatment
\<http://www.aafprs.org/patient/procedures/facial_scar.html\>

The AAFPRS site discusses making the decision to have skin resurfacing, types of procedures (Z-plasty, dermabrasion), and what to expect postsurgery; the focus is on scar revision of the face. Before/after illustrations are included.

American Society of Plastic Surgeons—Scar Revision
\<http://www.plasticsurgery.org/public_education/procedures/ScarRevision.cfm\>

The ASPS page on scar revision (see Figure 8.8) describes why you might consider this procedure, types of scars, risks of surgery, types of surgical procedures (Z-plasty, skin grafting, and flap surgery), and postsurgical information.

Facial Plastic Surgery Network—Scar Revision & Keloid Prevention
\<http://www.facialplasticsurgery.net/scar_revision.htm\>

This page can be reached directly via the URL, or go to the main page \<http://www.facialplasticsurgery.net\>, select "Facial Procedures," and then "Scar Revision/Keloid Prevention." This page is similar (whether you are a candidate for the procedure, procedure description, expectations, recovery, risks and complications, and more) to Yes They're Fake! (see as follows), but without the informal, chatty comments and product information.

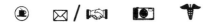

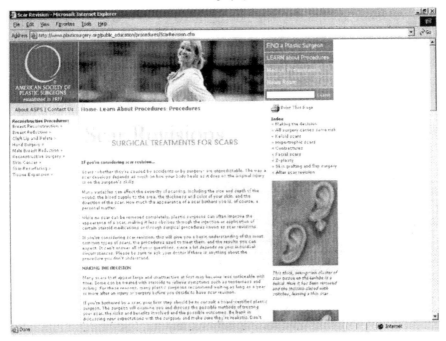

FIGURE 8.8. American Society of Plastic Surgeons—Scar Revision
<http://www.plasticsurgery.org/public_education/procedures/ScarRevision.cfm>

iEnhance—Scar Revision/Scar Repair
<http://www.ienhance.com/procedure/default.asp>

Go directly to the "Procedures" page and select either "Plastic Surgery" or "Facial Plastic Surgery," then under "Head/Face" select "Scar Revision/Scar Repair." The page includes basic information on the benefits of this surgery, options for surgical procedure, risks, postsurgical recovery, the ideal candidate for the procedure, and questions to ask your doctor. Procedures for scar revision include collagen injections, dermabrasion, laser skin resurfacing, punch grafting, tissue expansion, Z-plasty, and more.

Yes They're Fake!—Scar Revision
<http://www.yestheyrefake.net/scar_revision.htm>

This is a refreshingly candid site, created by a patient who has undergone cosmetic surgery herself. Go directly to the URL, or go to the main page <http://www.yestheyrefake.net>, select "Facial Procedures," and then "Scar Revision." The page describes scar revision, whether you are a candidate for the procedure, preoperative information, how the procedure is performed, the recovery, contraindications, and risks and complications.

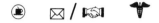

SCLEROTHERAPY

Spider veins (more technically called telangiectasias), are those small red, purple, or blue veins that appear on the thigh or lower leg, but can be located elsewhere on the body. They are broken veins or capillaries that can be removed without causing harm.

Sclerotherapy is the most frequently used treatment for spider veins. A sclerosing solution (saline—salt solution) is injected into the vein with a small needle; multiple injections are needed for each session. The solution causes the vein to collapse and gradually disappear. Spider veins in the facial area are usually treated with lasers instead of sclerotherapy.

2003 statistics:

ASAPS:	444,416	(431,257 in women)
ASPS:	482,575	(472,347 in women)

American Academy of Cosmetic Surgery—Sclerotherapy (Veins)
<http://www.cosmeticsurgery.org/procedures/sclerotherapy_vein_ surgery_.asp?mn=pc>

Go directly to the URL, or select "Patient Center," then "Learn About a Cosmetic Procedure," then "Sclerotherapy." The page contains basic information about spider veins, the procedure of sclerotherapy, post-surgery information, and risks. For costs, you are referred to your cosmetic surgeon.

American Academy of Dermatology—Spider Vein, Varicose Vein Therapy
<http://www.aad.org/public/Publicationspamphlets/Spidervein.htm>

This AAD pamphlet describes spider veins, their prevention and treatment. The primary treatment described in this pamphlet is sclerotherapy, although laser treatment is among several additional procedures mentioned.

American Society for Aesthetic Plastic Surgery—Sclerotherapy
<http://www.surgery.org/public/procedures-sclerotherapy.php>

This ASAPS page on sclerotherapy, the treatment for spider veins, describes the technique, benefits, and other considerations.

American Society for Dermatologic Surgery—Spider and Varicose Veins
<http://www.asds.net/Patients/FactSheets/patients-Fact_Sheet-veins.html>

Go directly to the URL, or select "Patients," then "Fact Sheets," and then "Spider and Varicose Veins." This ASDS fact sheet talks about spider and varicose veins and then focuses on sclerotherapy as the "gold standard" treatment for spider veins. Other treatments (laser surgery, electrodesiccation, surgical ligation and stripping, and ambulatory phlebectomy) are mentioned.

American Society of Plastic Surgeons—Sclerotherapy (Spider Veins)
<http://www.plasticsurgery.org/public_education/procedures/sclerotherapy.cfm>

This ASPS page on spider veins (sclerotherapy) includes a description of spider veins, candidates for surgery, a description of the treatment, along with risks and what to expect from the procedure.

iEnhance—Spider Vein Treatment (Sclerotherapy)
<http://www.ienhance.com/procedure/default.asp>

Go directly to the "Procedures" page and select "Plastic Surgery," then under "Legs" select "Spider Vein Treatment (Sclerotherapy)." The page (see Figure 8.9) includes basic information about spider veins, but focuses on sclerotherapy, the primary surgical procedure for spider veins, including risks, postsurgical recovery, the ideal candidate for the procedure, and questions to ask your doctor. A link is available to "laser treatment," which can also be used for spider veins.

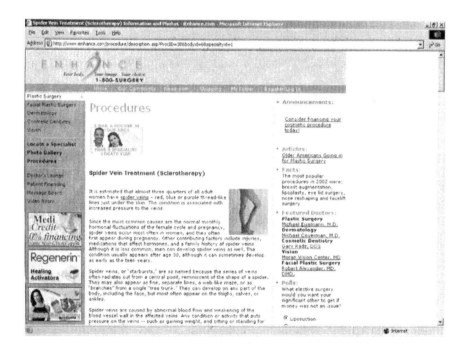

FIGURE 8.9. iEnhance—Spider Vein Treatment (Sclerotherapy) <http://www.ienhance.com/procedure/description.asp?ProcID=36&bodyid=6& specialtyid=1>
Reprinted with permission of iEnhance.com.

Medem—Spider Veins
<http://www.medem.com>

Input "Spider Veins" into the Medem search feature to locate this page. Information on spider veins is provided by the American Society of Plastic Surgeons, and discusses what spider veins are, along with the treatment, sclerotherapy.

SKIN MANAGEMENT

See WRINKLE TREATMENT (in this chapter). *See also* BOTULINUM TOXIN (BOTOX) INJECTIONS, CHEMICAL PEELS, DERMABRASION, INJECTABLE FILLERS, LASER SKIN RESURFACING, and SKIN RESURFACING (all in this chapter).

SKIN RESURFACING

Skin resurfacing smooths and refinishes the skin by removing blemishes, fine wrinkles, and other surface irregularities, resulting in a younger look. Methods used for skin resurfacing include chemical peels, dermabrasion, and laser resurfacing, each of which have their own section in this chapter. This section includes sites that review skin resurfacing as a whole. *See also* CHEMICAL PEELS, DERMABRASION, and LASER SKIN RESURFACING (in this chapter).

American Academy of Facial Plastic and Reconstructive Surgery— Understanding Skin Resurfacing
<http://www.aafprs.org/patient/procedures/resurfacing.html>

The AAFPRS site discusses the decision to have skin resurfacing, types of procedures (chemical peel, dermabrasion, laser surgery), and what to expect postsurgery; includes before/after illustrations.

American Society for Aesthetic Plastic Surgery—Skin Resurfacing
<http://www.surgery.org/public/procedures-skinresurface.php>

This ASAPS public page on skin resurfacing (see Figure 8.10), a technique used primarily on the face, leads to additional pages containing information about the surgical procedure, risks, before and after surgery, and more. This is one of the better sites available about skin resurfacing.

American Society of Plastic Surgeons—Skin Resurfacing
<http://www.plasticsurgery.org/public_education/procedures/
SkinResurfacing.cfm>

Although this ASPS page is listed as skin resurfacing, it is specifically focused on laser skin resurfacing. Included is information about what the

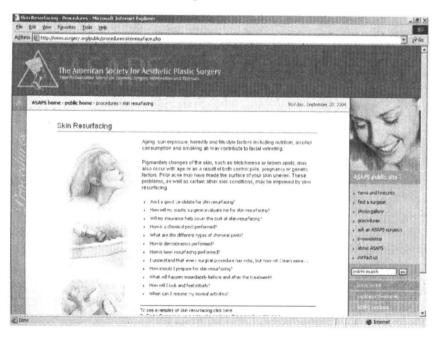

FIGURE 8.10. American Society for Aesthetic Plastic Surgery—Skin Resurfacing
<http://www.surgery.org/public/procedures-skinresurface.php>
Reprinted with permission of American Society for Aesthetic Plastic Surgery.

treatment is used for, a description of the procedure, best candidates for the procedure, risks, and what to expect from the procedure. The ASPS also has a separate page for "Laser Skin Resurfacing."

SOFT TISSUE FILLERS

See INJECTABLE FILLERS (in this chapter).

SPIDER VEINS

See LASER TREATMENT OF SPIDER VEINS and SCLEROTHERAPY (both in this chapter).

TATTOO REMOVAL

Tattoos can be removed with laser surgery, dermabrasion, or surgically; your physician will recommend the best treatment. *See also* DERMA-BRASION and LASER SKIN RESURFACING (both in this chapter).

American Society for Dermatologic Surgery—Tattoo Removal
<http://www.asds.net/Patients/FactSheets/patients-Fact_Sheet-tattoo_removal.html>

Go directly to the URL, or select "Patients," then "Fact Sheets," and then "Tattoo Removal." The ASDS fact sheet about tattoo removal includes information about tattoos, the procedures used to remove them (laser surgery, dermabrasion, surgical excision), and side effect/complication information.

Facial Plastic Surgery Network—Tattoo Removal
<http://www.facialplasticsurgery.net/tattoo_removal.htm>

This page can be reached directly via the URL, or go to the main page <http://www.facialplasticsurgery.net>, select "Facial Procedures," and then "Tattoo Removal." This page is similar (what is tattoo removal, whether you are a candidate for the procedure, procedure description, recovery, risks and complications, and more) to Yes They're Fake! (see as follows).

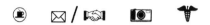

iEnhance—Tattoo Removal
<http://www.ienhance.com/procedure/default.asp>

Go directly to the "Procedures" page and select either "Plastic Surgery" or "Facial Plastic Surgery," then under "Head/Face" select "Tattoo Removal." The page (see Figure 8.11) includes basic information such as sur-

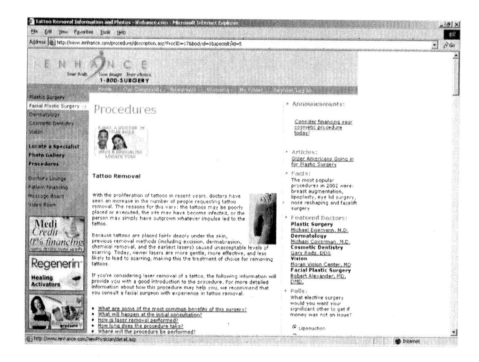

FIGURE 8.11. iEnhance—Tattoo Removal
<http://www.ienhance.com/procedure/description.asp?ProcID=17&bodyid=1&specialtyid=5>
Reprinted with permission of iEnhance.com.

gical procedure (laser removal), risks, postsurgical recovery, the ideal candidate for the procedure, and questions to ask your doctor.

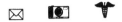

Yes They're Fake!—Tattoo Removal
<http://www.yestheyrefake.net/tattoo_removal.html>

This is a refreshingly candid site, created by a patient who has undergone cosmetic surgery herself. Go directly to the URL, or go to the main page <http://www.yestheyrefake.net>, select "Body Procedures," and then "Tattoo Removal." The page covers options in tattoo removal, preoperative information, how the procedure is performed, the recovery, contraindications, and risks and complications.

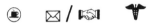

WRINKLE TREATMENT

Wrinkles develop over time and are primarily a result of aging. The sites included in this section review the various treatments for aging skin, from over-the-counter creams and lotions to Botox, skin resurfacing, and dermabrasion. *See also* other procedures such as BOTULINUM TOXIN (BOTOX) INJECTIONS, CHEMICAL PEELS, DERMABRASION, INJECTABLE FILLERS, and LASER SKIN RESURFACING (all in this chapter).

American Academy of Dermatology—Facial Skin Rejuvenation
<http://www.aad.org/public/Publications/pamphlets/
FacialSkinRejuvenation.htm>

This AAD pamphlet describes the general process of aging skin and procedures that might be used for rejuvenation, including topical products, fillers, chemical peels, dermabrasion, laser resurfacing, liposuction, and surgery. Treatment of each topic is brief, as this document is an overview. A related pamphlet is "Mature Skin" <http://www.aad.org/public/Publications/pamphlets/MatureSkin.htm>.

American Academy of Facial Plastic and Reconstructive Surgery—Understanding Wrinkle Treatment
<http://www.aafprs.org/patient/procedures/wrinkles.html>

This AAFPRS page describes the various treatments for removing wrinkles from the face (including Botox, injectable collagen, synthetic implants); it also discusses which treatment to choose, or combining these treatments with another surgical procedure, and what to expect after the treatment. Includes before/after illustrations.

American Society of Plastic Surgeons—Skin Management (Surface-Repair Treatments)
<http://www.plasticsurgery.org/public_education/procedures/SkinManagement.cfm>

This ASPS page on skin management covers the nonsurgical procedures of Retin-A and glycolic acid treatments. Included is a description of these two treatments, best candidates for the treatments, reactions/side effects, and posttreatment information.

Yes They're Fake!—Wrinkles
<http://www.yestheyrefake.net/wrinkle_improvement.html>

This is a refreshingly candid site, created by a patient who has undergone cosmetic surgery herself. Go directly to the URL, or go to the main page <http://www.yestheyrefake.net>, select "Facial Procedures," and then "Wrinkles." The page on wrinkles covers everything from over-the-counter lotions and creams to implants, Botox, chemical peels, and microdermabrasion.

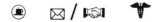

Chapter 9

Hair Transplantation for Women

Hair replacement surgery is not just for men! In fact, many sites on the Internet are including special sections about hair replacement surgery for women as they have "discovered" this new, expanded market for permanent hair replacement. This chapter covers hair replacement surgery; although some sites will list nonsurgical methods of treating hair loss, the focus is on hair transplantation.

Women tend to lose hair differently than men; the loss is often diffuse—a generalized loss throughout the scalp. However, some women experience patches of hair loss similar to men, including balding on the crown of the head and thinning at the front of the hairline. A recent article has attempted to classify hair loss in women.[1] Hair loss in women can be due to hormone changes, aging, stress, diet, and a variety of medical reasons, including thyroid disease. In addition, permanent hair loss in women may occur from chemotherapy or radiotherapy (e.g., from cancer therapy), or damage may occur around the hairline due to other cosmetic surgical procedures. For many women, hair transplantation offers a better solution than temporary or inconvenient "fixes" to cover hair loss.

All of these reasons factor into why more and more women are deciding to undergo hair replacement surgery, rather than using nonsurgical methods such as wigs and hair extensions to cover hair loss, or the constant application of medications such as minoxidil (Rogaine) to stimulate hair growth. The American Society of Plastic Surgeons indicates that in 2003, 12 percent, or 3,751 of 31,737 hair transplants performed by their member physicians were for women; the American Society for Aesthetic Plastic Surgery statistics for 2003 show that 10.5 percent of hair transplantations were performed on female patients. However, the Web sites of many physicians' practices indicate that women make up to 40 percent of their business.

Hair restoration treatments range from use of drugs such as Rogaine to hair extensions to hair transplantation. Many of the clinics that perform these procedures utilize technicians and laypeople; physicians are used to perform occasional surgical procedures. You should be aware that there is no board certification for hair transplantation. Instead, you can expect your surgeon to be board certified in a variety of specialties, from plastic surgery to dermatology. A board certified physician who specializes in liposuction and body contouring but also performs occasional hair transplantation may not be the proper specialist for you. If you decide that hair transplantation is the right decision for you, you should look not only at the doctor's credentials, but his or her experience in hair transplantation. For instance, how many transplants does he or she perform per year; how long has he or she been performing transplants; and, is it the primary procedure that he or she performs? Ask to see examples of the doctor's work. Your physician should be willing to answer all of these questions to help you make your decision.

The Internet is overloaded with sites about hair loss—especially "miracle" cures proclaiming to stop hair loss, alternative forms of treatments, and special products. The sources listed in this chapter represent carefully selected sites recommended as sources to begin your search about hair transplantation. These include noncommercial sites such as organizations, associations, and government sites. The purpose of most hair restoration commercial sites is to introduce you to their services, i.e., to get you to contact them and make an appointment. However, many of these sites have excellent information, whether or not you choose to use the doctors/ services listed on their site. This select list includes examples of private practices, group practices, and physician locator services. Listing of a commercial site is not an endorsement of products, "locator" services, or physicians. Rather, these commercial sites were selected for one of two reasons: the site has a large amount of quality information about female hair loss, or the Web site is well done and subscribes to the HONcode principles.

HAIR TRANSPLANTATION SITES

American Academy of Dermatology—Hair Restoration
<http://www.aad.org/public/Publications/pamphlets/HairRestoration. htm>

The AAD page on hair restoration covers the topic for both women and men. It offers basic information about the causes and types of hair loss, who makes a good candidate for hair restoration surgery, types of surgical treatments and options, and possible complications.

American Academy of Facial Plastic and Reconstructive Surgery— Understanding Hair Replacement Surgery
<http://www.aafprs.org>

The AAFPRS site has basic information about hair loss and hair replacement surgery, including what to expect postsurgery. According to the AAFPRS, hair loss affects "one in five women." Information here is applicable to both men and women. The physician finder has an extensive list of board-certified physicians, but keep in mind that the surgeon may specialize in areas other than hair transplantation.

American Board of Hair Restoration Surgery
<http://www.abhrs.com>

This site contains a "Directory of Diplomates," searchable by state and physician name, of physicians certified by the ABHRS. The list of certified physicians is extremely small. Contains no other information for prospective patients.

American Hair Loss Council
<http://www.ahlc.org>

The American Hair Loss Council is a nonprofit membership organization of persons interested in treatment for hair loss, from cosmetologists and barbers through dermatologists. The AHLC certifies nonphysician hair loss specialists. The site includes nonbiased information about both surgical and nonsurgical treatments. From the home page, select "What causes hair loss?" and then "Female Pattern Hair Loss" or go directly to <http://www.ahlc.org/causes-f.htm> to find the page specific to hair loss in women—"Androgenetic Alopecia (Female Pattern Hair Loss)." The site has a "Find a Specialist in Your Area," which will be available in the near future.

American Osteopathic College of Dermatology—Female Pattern Hair Loss
<http://www.aocd.org/skin/dermatologic_diseases/female_pattern_hai.html>

This site has a basic description of androgenetic alopecia, or female pattern hair loss, and includes treatment information from Rogaine through transplantation.

American Society for Aesthetic Plastic Surgery—Hair Transplantation
<http://surgery.org/public/procedures-hairtrans.asp>

The ASAPS procedure page on hair transplantation covers basic hair transplant techniques, benefits, and other considerations. The site is not specific to women's hair loss, but useful. The "Find a Surgeon" feature allows you to locate a surgeon either inside or outside the United States, but keep in mind that the surgeon may not specialize in hair transplantation.

American Society for Dermatologic Surgery—Hair Restoration Treatments
<http://www.asds.net/Patients/FactSheets/patients-Fact_Sheet-hair_rest.html>

The ASDS fact sheet has general information about hair restoration, including surgical and nonsurgical techniques. It is not specific to women's hair loss, but useful. "Find a Derm Surgeon" links to an extensive list of dermatology certified surgeons, specialists in all areas of dermatologic surgery, and also allows you to limit your search to surgeons who perform hair transplantation.

American Society of Plastic Surgeons—Hair Replacement
<http://www.plasticsurgery.org/public_education/procedures/
  HairReplacement.cfm>

The ASPS public information page on hair replacement includes "best candidates" for hair replacement, a description of the surgery, risks, post-surgical recovery, and before/after illustrations. Included is information about hair loss in women. "Find a Plastic Surgeon" allows you to locate an ASPS member near you (not specific to hair transplants); you can look for either a cosmetic or reconstructive surgeon.

eMedicine—Hair Replacement Surgery, Hair Transplantation
  in Women
<http://www.emedicine.com/plastic/topic523.htm>

This is an article by Dr. Mark E. Krugman, a clinical professor at the University of California at Irvine School of Medicine. It covers the hair transplantation procedure, the etiology of hair loss in women, and has an extensive photo gallery.

Hair Loss Patient Guide
<http://www.hairlosspatientguide.com>

This site has everything from general hair loss information to the transplant procedure and post-op issues. It has a page specific to wo-men, "Hair Loss and Hair Restoration in Women," at <http://www.hairlosspatientguide.com/female_hair_loss.html>. Only an e-mail address is given for contact information; however, many of the pages are provided courtesy of the Physician's Hair Transplant Institute, Inc., and clicking on that link takes you to the site of a hair transplant group, International Hair Transplant Institute (which is listed separately in this chapter).

Hair Loss Research—Hair Transplantation in Women
<http://www.hairlossresearch.com/hair_transplant_articles/jepstein_women.htm>

This is a detailed article, "Hair Transplantation in Women: Treating Female Pattern Hair Loss and Repairing the Distortion and Scarring from Prior Cosmetic Surgery," by Dr. Jeffrey S. Epstein, a physician in private practice in Miami, Florida. The paper gives detailed information about the technique of hair transplantation in female patients for both female pattern hair loss and hair loss caused by facial cosmetic surgery. The paper is fairly technical but provides extensive, descriptive information not included on most other Internet sites.

Hair Loss Scams!
<http://www.hairlossscams.com>

This site, made available by DermMatch, Inc. (makers of DermMatch Topical Shading, one of the recommended products on this site), offers ways to spot a hair loss scam and government agencies to contact about scams (e.g., FDA and FTC), with links included. Hair loss resources (books, Web sites, professional organizations) are also given. Keep in mind that even this site is not free of bias because of its commercial sponsorship.

Hair Loss Specialists—Female Hair Loss
<http://www.hairlossspecialists.com/forwomen.cfm>

This site has extensive information about hair loss in women, including causes of hair loss, differences between hair loss in women and men, treatment options, transplant surgery, a photo gallery, FAQs, and more. The doctor finder feature locates nationwide offices of Medical Hair Restoration, a private company, so this site is included for the information, rather than as a physician locator.

Hair Replacement Surgery
\<http://www.hairtransplantation.com\>

This is the page of Dr. John Kiely, a hair transplant surgeon who is located in Maryland. It is an example of quality information that can be found on the Web site of a practicing physician. The site has excellent information about causes of hair loss, new advances in the treatment of hair loss, FAQs, and options to hair transplantation. Notable is a special section "For Women" (click on this section from the main page or go directly to \<http://www.hairtransplantation.com/women.html\>), plus an article, "Incidence of Female Androgenetic Alopecia" \<http://www.hairtransplantation. com/advances/incidence.html\> (or, select "Medical Advances," then "Archives" and then the article).

Hair Transplant Adviser
\<http://www.hairtransplantadviser.org\>

Despite this being listed as an organization (.org), it is a private site. The goal of the site is to help you "make the best possible choices in dealing with your hair loss." In addition to basic information on hair loss and hair transplantation, the site offers advice about realistic expectations, finding quality care, and tries to dispel some myths about hair transplantation. Follicular unit transplantation is emphasized as the preferred transplant method. A strength of the site is an extensive list of links. The International Alliance of Hair Restoration Surgeons is used as the physician locator service.

Hair Transplant Medical
\<http://www.hairtransplantmedical.com\>

This site has everything from the basics of hair growth and hair loss to treatments (e.g., medications, hair transplantation, alternative therapies). "Hair Transplant 101" includes "What is a Hair Transplant," "Are you a Candidate?" and "Questions to ask your doctor" while "Beyond the Basics" has more in-depth topics such as "Bad Hair Transplants—Repair" and "When to be Suspicious." The site uses the International Alliance of Hair Restoration Surgeons as its physician "locator" service, searchable by physician or state (of limited use because of the small number of physicians). Also included is "Women and Hair Transplants" <http://www.hairtransplantmedical.com/women/index.htm>. The site also includes article reprints from professional journals (one specific to women). Links to other sites provide additional resources. Although Hair Transplant Medical is a consumer organization, it is, in fact, a physician locator site that also provides consumer information. A drawback to this site is that its "owner" could not be identified, other than the comment, "Please note that I am not a doctor, so I cannot provide you any advice for your hair loss," plus an e-mail address. The site suffers from multiple typographical errors.

Hair Transplant Network
<http://www.hairtransplantnetwork.com>

The Hair Transplant Network offers a variety of information on hair transplantation in general, and some specific information related to hair loss and hair restoration in women. Included are before-and-after photos; basic information on hair restoration and transplantation, hair transplant articles (research library), a discussion group, and physician referral (at the time of evaluation, forty-five doctors were listed worldwide). In addition to reading the general information, women should do a site search on "women" or "female" to bring up several interesting articles specific to hair loss, transplantation, and restoration in women. The site offers other features such as a discussion group, FAQs, and "Find a 'Mentor.'"

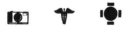

International Alliance of Hair Restoration Surgeons
<http://www.iahrs.org>

The IAHRS "is a consumer organization that selectively screens skilled and ethical hair transplant surgeons." This site includes the organization's mission, code of ethics, misconduct information, and FAQs, along with members and a "Find a Doctor" service, plus a service to inquire about credentials of the doctor who performed your hair transplantation. Links are available to members' Web sites. This is a small, but growing organization in a field that does not have "official" board certification. Members of this organization must perform follicular unit hair transplantations, "prove their surgical skill and artistic ability," and "agree to impromptu inspections of their surgical facilities."

International Hair Transplant Institute
<http://www.forhair.com>

This is the site of the hair transplant group led by Dr. John P. Cole, who operates multiple sites in the United States and affiliate sites in Europe. The site contains information about the transplant procedure, a "live chat" link, and a patient guide (eighty-one-page PDF download) on hair restoration (Chapter 16 is devoted to women). This site contains contact information for prospective patients of this transplant group practice.

International Society of Hair Restoration Surgery
<http://www.ishrs.org>

The ISHRS is a membership organization of hair restoration specialists with a mission of advancing "the art and science of hair restoration by licensed, experienced physicians." This site contains a wealth of information on the reasons for hair loss and both surgical and nonsurgical treatments of hair loss. Included are special considerations such as hair restorations in ethnic/minority groups, FAQs, and patient experiences. The easiest way to locate information about hair loss in women is to go to the "Site Map" and scan articles for "women" or "female." Pages of special interest to women include "Hair Loss and Restoration in Women" <http://www.ishrs.org/articles/hair-loss-women.htm>, "Hair Transplants are for Women Too" <http://www.ishrs.org/articles/hairtransplants-women.htm>, and "Hair Loss and Female Pattern Baldness" <http://www.ishrs.org/hair-loss/hair-loss-female.htm>. Also included is the "Find a Doctor" feature that helps you locate a member of ISHRS near you; the listing includes about 700 specialists worldwide. In addition to address and phone information, many of the doctor profiles include e-mail addresses and Web sites for further information. The ISHRS site should be among the first to visit when looking for basic hair transplantation information.

MedlinePlus—Medical Encyclopedia—Female Pattern Baldness
<http://www.nlm.nih.gov/medlineplus/ency/article/001173.htm>

This page on "Female Pattern Baldness" from the Medical Encyclopedia in MedlinePlus links to sites with basic information about causes, symptoms, and treatment for female pattern baldness, including medication, hair transplants, and hair pieces (see Figure 9.1).

New Hair Institute
<http://www.newhair.com>

New Hair Institute (NHI) "is the pioneer of Follicular Unit Hair Transplantation and Follicular Unit Extraction." "NHI is a medical group of board certified physicians devoted solely to hair restoration." The NHI site contains basic information on hair transplantation, and an extensive explanation of FUT and FUE. Extensive information on "Hair Loss in Women" can be found at <http://newhair.com/resources/women.asp>. The site promotes this medical group's services, which has several locations, and includes a video gallery, physician information, fees, and consultation/appointment services.

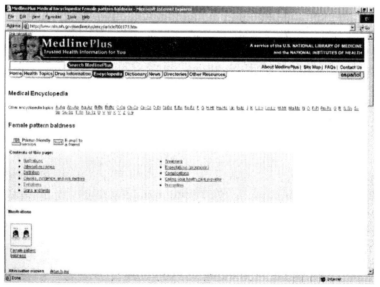

FIGURE 9.1. MedlinePlus—Medical Encyclopedia—Female Pattern Baldness
<http://www.nlm.nih.gov/medlineplus/ency/article/001173.htm>

Regrowth.com
<http://www.regrowth.com/female_hair_loss.cfm>

Despite this site's very commercial look, with ads placed throughout many of its pages, the content is easy to read and fairly neutral (nonsurgical treatments are preferred). The site was founded in 1996 and is still edited by Mr. John Ertel, who searched the Internet for his own hair loss problem and "was unable to find a comprehensive site that provided objective information." He decided to create his own Web site, which led to the Regrowth Network (Regrowth.com), which includes the set of commercial and noncommercial links from the "Hair Loss Sites" page. This site has information about hair loss and treatments (both surgical and nonsurgical), chat groups and forums, and much more. In addition to general information about hair loss, for information specific to women, select "Regrowth for Women" from the home page or go directly to <http://www.regrowth.com/female_hair_loss.cfm> (see Figure 9.2). The women's section includes information on "Causes of Hair Loss," the "Female Hair Loss Scale," "Diagnosis," "Hair Transplantation," "Non-Surgical Hair Replacement," and "Discussion Forums." The "Women's Forum" offers a "support forum for female members experiencing hair loss."

Virtual Hospital—Hair Transplants: Frequently Asked Questions
<http://www.vh.org/adult/patient/surgery/faq/hairtransplant.html>

The Virtual Hospital's page on hair transplants is presented as FAQs as presented to and answered by Dr. Albert Cram, a physician at the University of Iowa, which produces the Virtual Hospital. Several questions are specific to female hair loss.

WebMD—Hair Loss Solutions for Women
<http://my.webmd.com/content/article/79/95994.html>

In WebMD, a search for "hair loss in women" links to the page, "Hair Loss Solutions for Women" (go to the direct link, or go to <http://webmd.com> and use the search box). This page includes information on the emotional impact that hair loss has on women, and has links to "Treatments That Work," "Alternative Solutions" (diet and supplements), and "Hair Transplants for Women?"

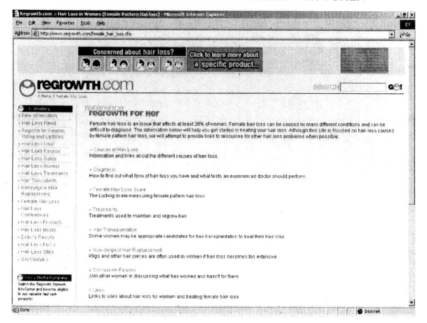

FIGURE 9.2. Regrowth for Women
<http://www.regrowth.com/female_hair_loss.cfm>
Reprinted with permission of Regrowth.com.

Women With Hair Loss
<http://www.womenwithhairloss.com>

This site is directed at meeting "the challenges of women suffering from hair loss." The site has an extensive FAQs page, a message board and chat rooms, and a specialist search (based on physician practices that have signed up with this service). Despite its commercial nature (there is a page of products for sale and information for physicians joining the service), quite a bit of useful information related specifically to women's hair loss can be found here.

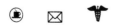

NOTE

1. Vogel, James E. "Hair Transplantation in Women: A Practical New Classification System and Review of Technique." *Aesthetic Surgery Journal* 22(2002): 247-259.

Chapter 10

Cosmetic Dentistry

Cosmetic dentistry is an area that has gained prominence recently, partly due to its use in TV programs such as *Extreme Makeover* and *The Swan,* where dental work is done along with other cosmetic procedures. The American Academy of Cosmetic Dentistry, founded in 1984, offers accreditation and fellowship programs that provide "postgraduate and certification in cosmetic dentistry to both dentists and laboratory technicians." As new techniques and methods for improving the appearance of teeth continue to be developed, this dental specialization seems poised to increase in popularity.

Treatments include whitening, bonding, dental implants, crowns, and veneers. Many procedures that are considered to be "cosmetic" can be done routinely in a dentist's office. Other procedures are more specialized, but your dentist will know who offers these cosmetic procedures in your area. If you are interested in improving the appearance of your teeth, it is important to become familiar with what cosmetic dental procedures are available and what might be appropriate for your needs.

Because each of the sites includes descriptions of almost all cosmetic dental procedures, this chapter is not divided by procedure, but is organized alphabetically by the name of the site. Several specialties recognized by the American Dental Association may be involved with cosmetic procedures and are listed among these sites. Information about cosmetic dentistry applies equally to women and men.

COSMETIC DENTISTRY SITES

Academy of General Dentistry—Consumer Information
\<http://www.agd.org/consumer/index.html\>

The Academy of General Dentistry (AGD) is a membership organization of over 37,000 general dentists. They bill their Web site as the "'go to' dental resource for the general practitioner—and the organization for consumers to find reliable oral health information." From the "Consumer Information" page, you can link to "50 oral health topics," "Find a Dentist," and a message board. Among the oral health topics are: "Cosmetics," "Bleaching," "Crowns," "Implants," and "Veneers." Each of these pages then links to articles about the specific topic, for example, "Cosmetics" links to several articles, including "Improving Your Smile"; while "Veneers" links to articles such as "What are Porcelain Veneers?" "Dental Terms" links to brief definitions of dental terminology.

Aetna InteliHealth
\<http://www.intelihealth.com\>

InteliHealth is a quality consumer health site, with information primarily provided by the Harvard Medical School. The dental portion is provided by the University of Pennsylvania School of Dental Medicine. Selecting "Dental Health" takes you to a commercial site, "Simple Steps to Better Dental Health" \<http://www.simplestepsdental.com\>, which is detailed later in this chapter.

American Academy of Cosmetic Dentistry
\<http://www.aacd.com\>

The American Academy of Cosmetic Dentistry (AACD) is "the world's largest organization of cosmetic dental professionals." Founded in 1984, the AACD "is dedicated to advancing the art and science of cosmetic dentistry." The AACD site (see Figure 10.1) is a great starting place for information about cosmetic dentistry. From the main page, in the "For the Public" section, you can link directly to "Find a Cosmetic Dentist," "About Cosmetic Dentistry, "AACD Smile Gallery," and "Patient Literature." Or, by clicking on "For the Public," you are taken to a page \<http://www.

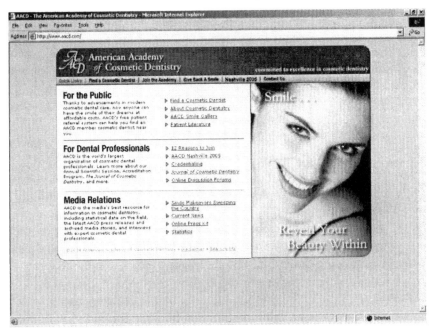

FIGURE 10.1. American Academy of Cosmetic Dentistry Home Page
<http://www.aacd.com>
Reprinted with permission of American Academy of Cosmetic Dentistry.

aacd.com/public/default.aspx> that gives additional choices, including "AACD Extreme Makeover doctors" and a multimedia presentation. Additional links can be found by "mousing over" links on the top bar; you can find a glossary of terms, brief descriptions of procedures, and more extensive brochures on "The Art of Veneers," "The Art of Whitening," and "Your Smile Says it All!" This site has a cosmetic dentist finder. Also included is information for the media and for dental professionals.

American Academy of Periodontology
<http://www.perio.org>

The American Academy of Periodontology is one of nine specialty organizations recognized by the American Dental Association. This specialty deals with "the prevention, diagnosis and treatment of diseases affecting the gums and supporting structures of the teeth and in the placement and maintenance of dental implants." From the left-hand section, "For the Public," choose articles on "Dental Implants for Tooth Replacement," "Plastic Surgery to Enhance Your Smile" (periodontal plastic procedures), and periodontal procedures (includes dental implants and cosmetic procedures). Or, from the menu bar near the top of the main page, "mouse over" "Public" and select from the pop-ups. Clicking "Public" from this menu bar takes you to the consumer page <http://www.perio. org/consumer/index.html>, which basically has the same information available from the main page. You can also locate a local periodontist via this site.

American Association of Orthodontists—Public Information
<http://www.braces.org>

Orthodontics, one of the nine specialties recognized by the American Dental Association, "is the branch of dentistry that specializes in the diagnosis, prevention and treatment of dental and facial irregularities." Orthodontists correct the bite, alignment and spacing of teeth. From the main page, select "About Orthodontics" and then use links to connect to "Facts about Orthodontics," "Considering Orthodontic Treatment?" and more. Local orthodontists can be located via this site.

American College of Prosthodontists
<http://www.prosthodontics.org>

Prosthodontists are "specialists in the restoration and replacement of teeth." They specialize in restoring "function and esthetics to your smile" with procedures such as crowns, bridges, inlays, dentures, veneers, and dental implants. The American College of Prosthodontists is one of nine specialties recognized by the American Dental Association. From the main ACP page, select "Consumers/Patients" and then link to "Find a Prosthodontist," "Improve Your Smile," "Consumer FAQ's," a photo gallery, and more.

American Dental Association
<http://www.ada.org>

The American Dental Association (ADA) "is the professional association of dentists committed to the public's health, ethics, science and professional advancement." On the ADA page, under "Your Oral Health," select "A-Z Topics." Topics include "Cosmetic Dentistry," "Bridges," "Crowns," "Tooth Whitening Treatments," and "Veneers." Also available in "Your Oral Health" are "Frequently Asked Questions (FAQs)" and "Tips for Finding a Dentist." On the "A-Z Topics" page is a link to a very useful "Glossary of Terms" (left side of the page). This site has a dentist search feature, "Find an ADA Member Dentist."

Canadian Dental Association—Cosmetic Dentistry
<http://www.cda-adc.ca/English/your_oral_health/dental_ procedures/cosmetic/default.asp>

Go directly to the URL, or, from the CDA main page, select "Your Oral Health," then "Dental Procedures," and then "Cosmetic Dentistry." This page contains basic information about teeth whitening, bonding, and veneers, and describes the procedures and materials used, along with what results to expect. This site is also available in French.

Facial Plastic Surgery Network—Cosmetic Dentistry
<http://www.facialplasticsurgery.net/cosmetic_dentistry.htm>

This page can be reached directly via the URL, or go to the main page <http://www.facialplasticsurgery.net>, select "Facial Procedures," and then "Cosmetic Dental." This page is similar (orthodontics, tooth whitening, porcelain veneers and crowns, and gums) to Yes They're Fake! (see as follows), but without the informal, chatty comments.

iEnhance—Cosmetic Dentistry
<http://www.ienhance.com/speciality/dentistry.asp>

This page (see Figure 10.2) links to "Cosmetic Dentistry" (*sic*—speciality in URL), from which you can find a cosmetic dental specialist, go to the photo gallery, learn about cosmetic procedures, and ask questions of a cosmetic dentist. Or, you can go directly to the list of cosmetic procedures at <http://www.ienhance.com/procedures/procedure_list.asp?SpecialtyID=3>. The procedures list on this site is perhaps the most comprehensive of the cosmetic dentistry sites, and includes composite bonding, crowns, tooth whitening, porcelain veneers, cerinate veneers, dental implants, tooth contouring, and more. For each topic, the procedure is described, along with what to expect afterward, "ideal" candidates, risks, approximate costs, questions to ask your dentist, and more.

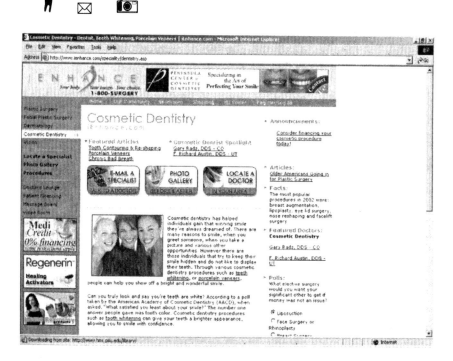

FIGURE 10.2. iEnhance—Cosmetic Dentistry
<http://www.ienhance.com/speciality/dentistry.asp>
Reprinted with permission of iEnhance.com.

MedlinePlus—Cosmetic Dentistry
<http://www.nlm.nih.gov/medlineplus/cosmeticdentistry.html>

The MedlinePlus site links you to quality Web sites about cosmetic dentistry (see Figure 10.3). MedlinePlus is produced by the National Library of Medicine specifically for patients and health care consumers, and is always an excellent place to begin your search.

Simple Steps to Better Dental Health
<http://www.simplestepsdental.com>

You can find this site via Aetna InteliHealth (listed earlier in this chapter), or go directly to the Simple Steps Web site. This site is jointly sponsored by Aetna and the University of Pennsylvania School of Dental Medicine. From this main page, select "Cosmetic Dentistry" (listed under "General Topics"), and then link to a variety of cosmetic dentistry topics—whitening, bonding, crown lengthening, veneers, recontouring, inlays,

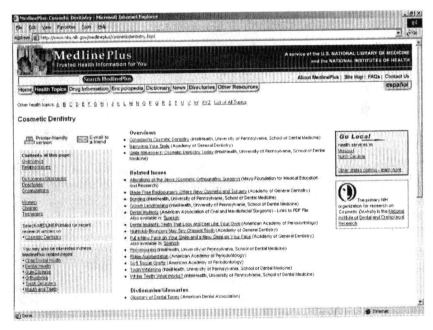

FIGURE 10.3. MedlinePlus—Cosmetic Dentistry
<http://www.nlm.nih.gov/medlineplus/cosmeticdentistry.html>

general information, and more. Transcripts are available from some of the chat sessions held at this site. Also of interest from "General Topics" are "Orthodontics" and "Periodontics."

WebMDHealth—Dental Health Center
<http://my.webmd.com/health_and_wellness/living_better/dental_ health_center/default.htm>

WebMD is a reliable health information provider and has fairly extensive information available about cosmetic dentistry in general, and about specific procedures such as teeth whitening, veneers, crowns, restorations, bonding, recontouring, and more. This information is provided in collaboration with the Cleveland Clinic. You can go directly to the "Dental Health Center" using the URL and then select "Cosmetic Dentistry" and then specific procedures; or, go to <http://www.webmd.com>, search for "Cosmetic Dentistry," choose the "Dental Health Center," and then "Cosmetic Dentistry." This site displays the HONcode.

Yes They're Fake!—Cosmetic Dentistry
<http://www.yestheyrefake.net/cosmetic_dental.html>

This refreshingly candid site was created by a patient who has undergone cosmetic surgery herself, and includes everything from over-the-counter whitening products (e.g., Crest Whitestrips), to professional whitening systems and laser whitening. Other cosmetic dentistry topics listed include orthodontics, porcelain crowns and veneers, bonding, and gum surgery. Average prices for dental procedures are given. You can access this information by going directly to the URL, or go to the main page <http://www.yestheyrefake.net>, select "Facial Procedures," and then "Cosmetic Dentistry."

✉ / 🤝 ⚕

Chapter 11

International Cosmetic Surgery Associations

Information in the previous chapters has been primarily from U.S. Web sites; readers from outside the United States will find much valuable information from these U.S. sites. However, excellent non-U.S. sources are also available that will be relevant and useful to both U.S. and non-U.S. readers who are considering cosmetic surgery. Cosmetic surgery, while becoming more commonplace in the United States, has been considered "routine" in many other countries for some time now. Worldwide, many people take vacations that incorporate cosmetic surgery and recovery time from the surgery.

The same methods of searching as mentioned earlier will apply—using a Web browser or directory to search for your topic, or going directly to a known URL. To point you in the right direction, selected sites are listed in this chapter. This list consists of non-U.S. professional associations specializing in cosmetic surgery and plastic surgery, and related medical specialties. It is not intended to be comprehensive and is weighted heavily toward English-speaking countries. Also, selected sites must have information intended for health consumers or patients; sites intended primarily for physicians are excluded.

Information provided by a professional association or society in your country (or the country in which you plan on having your surgery) is the best place to start. Web sites will usually give overview information for many procedures, indicate standards for member physicians, and provide a list of accredited cosmetic or plastic surgeons (some with links to the surgeons' Web sites). Web sites for international (including multinational) associations/organizations are listed first, followed by associations from specific countries. This list is representative, and offers but a sampling of cosmetic surgery organizations worldwide.

INTERNATIONAL/MULTINATIONAL ASSOCIATIONS

European Academy of Facial Plastic Surgery
<http://www.eafps.com>

Select "Patient Information" to get to information about procedures and a membership list searchable by name or country. The procedure information (eight procedures) is reprinted with permission from the American Academy of Facial Plastic and Reconstructive Surgery.

International Confederation for Plastic, Reconstructive and Aesthetic Surgery (IPRAS)
<http://www.ipras.org>

IPRAS promotes plastic surgery, both clinically and scientifically, worldwide. "Public Info" is limited to locating physicians in member countries.

International Society of Aesthetic Plastic Surgery
<http://www.isaps.org/>

This site is intended for the public to "provide it with information regarding organization and practice of Aesthetic Plastic Surgery all around the world." The site provides general information along with a list of qualified plastic surgeons and their home country.

PLink; The Plastic Surgery Links Collection
<http://www.nvpc.nl/plink>

This site, created by the Netherlands Society for Plastic Surgery, is a searchable database of links to sites on the Internet that deal with plastic surgery. Links are to doctors' sites, organizations, journals, and more, all related to plastic surgery; the site is searchable by subject. This is a great site to locate plastic surgery organizations by country.

World Plastic Surgery
<http://www.ipras.org/>

This site is maintained by the International Confederation for Plastic, Reconstructive and Aesthetic Surgery (IPRAS) and The International

Plastic, Reconstructive and Aesthetic Foundation (IPRAF) to provide information about plastic surgery for the general public.

COSMETIC SURGERY ASSOCIATIONS BY COUNTRY

Argentina

Sociedad Argentina de Cirugía Plástica, Estética y Reparadora (SACPER)
<http://www.sacper.org/ar/>

This site is in Spanish. Select "Procedimientos" for patient information about specific procedures; includes membership information (locate a physician).

Sociedad de Cirugía Plástica de Buenos Aires
<http://www.scpba.com.ar>

Available in Spanish and English. Both versions have "Surgeries" ("Cirugias"); more than twenty procedures are listed in the Spanish version, while the English version was still under construction. Selecting "Members" ("Miembros") gives an alphabetical list of members.

Australia

Australian Society of Plastic Surgeons
<http://www.plasticsurgery.org.au>

This site is the location for Australians to begin their search for plastic surgery information. Articles on a variety of procedures are available along with a database of society members searchable by location, name, and procedures. Also included are links to other associations and a list of FAQs.

Canada

Canadian Academy of Facial Plastic and Reconstructive Surgery
<http://www.facialcosmeticsurgery.org>

This site has a physician locator and information on surgical procedures (e.g., brow lift, rhinoplasty, otoplasty, hair restoration), nonsurgical cosmetic procedures (e.g., Botox, microdermabrasion, fat transfer), and a photo gallery, in addition to information for member physicians.

Canadian Laser Aesthetic Surgery Society (CLASS)
<http://www.class.ca/>

Locate a member, plus information on cosmetic procedures. Site is in English and French.

Canadian Society for Aesthetic (Cosmetic) Plastic Surgery
<http://www.csaps.ca>

The CSAPS site includes information about surgical procedures, along with a "Find a Surgeon" feature. This site can also be reached from the Canadian Society of Plastic Surgeons <http://www.plasticsurgery.ca> by selecting "Aesthetic Plastic Surgery Site." Information is available in English and French.

Canadian Society of Plastic Surgeons
<http://www.plasticsurgery.ca/>

This professional society seeks to advance the practice of cosmetic surgery. Enter the site by selecting English or French. Select "Surgeon Referral" to locate a plastic surgeon, "Procedures" for information about the most common plastic surgery procedures, or "Aesthetic Plastic Surgery Site" to take you to <http://www.csaps.ca> for further public information. Site is in English and French.

Cosmetic Surgery Canada
<http://cosmeticsurgerycanada.com/>

This is a commercial site that provides a surgeon search and referral service.

England (See Great Britain)

France

Société Francaise de Chirurgie Plastique Reconstructrice et Esthétique (SFCPRE)
<http://www.plasticiens.org>

Available in French. For a description of procedures, select "Interventions." Includes FAQs.

Société Francaise des Chirurgiens Esthétiques Plasticiens (French Society of Aesthetic Plastic Surgery)
<http://www.sofcep.org/>

Available in French. An English front-end page can be found at <http://www.sofcep.org/uk/index.htm>.

Germany

Vereinigung der deutschen Plastischen Chirurgen
<http://www.plastische-chirurgie.de/index2.html>

Available in German.

Great Britain

British Association of Aesthetic Plastic Surgeons (BAAPS)
<http://www.baaps.org.uk>

BAAPS was founded to advance "education in, and the practice of, aesthetic plastic surgery for public interest." This site includes a "Find a Surgeon" feature along with information about cosmetic procedures. Selecting "About Plastic Surgery" will provide qualifications and reasons to select a BAAPS member surgeon; provides descriptions of many plastic surgery procedures, and FAQs.

British Association of Plastic Surgeons
\<http://www.plastic-surgery.org.uk\>

"The Association is the professional representative body for plastic and reconstructive surgeons in the United Kingdom," and is therefore the recommended location for readers in Great Britain to begin their search for information. The site contains information on procedures and members.

British Society for Surgery of the Hand
\<http://www.bssh.ac.uk\>

Select "Resources," and then select from Patient Leaflets, Publications, Links, Members, and Support Groups.

Italy

Società Italiana di Chirurgia Plastica Ricostruttiva ed Estetica
\<http://www.sicpre.org\>

Available in Italian. Select "Interventi" for descriptions of procedures.

Mexico

Asociación Mexicana de Cirugía Plástica, Estética y Reconstructiva
\<http://www.cirugiaplastica.org.mx/\>

Available in Spanish. An English version is available at \<http://www.plasticsurgery.org.mx\>. The site includes information about selecting a qualified surgeon, and membership requirements; this site is primarily a directory of members.

Netherlands

Nederlandse Vereniging voor Plastische Chirurgie
\<http://www.nvpc.nl/nvpc/index.htm\>

Gives information on plastic surgery for both patients and doctors. This site is in Dutch. This site is the "home" of PLink (the Plastic Surgery Links Collection), an aggregator of plastic surgery information. PLink site is in English.

South Africa

Association of Plastic and Reconstructive Surgeons of Southern Africa
<http://www.plasticsurgeons.co.za>

Includes information on finding a plastic surgeon in South Africa along with "Overseas Visitors Information" for patients who are coming to South Africa for surgery. Brief patient information on procedures is available in "Questions and Answers" and "Articles of Interest," but this site relies on links to other organizations to provide more detailed information about plastic surgery procedures.

Spain

Sociedad Española de Cirugía Plástica, Reparadora y Estética (SECPRE)
<http://www.secpre.org>

Available in Spanish. Contains information for patients and a doctor locator.

Switzerland

Swiss Society of Plastic Reconstructive and Aesthetic Surgery (Societe Suisse Chirurgie Plastique, Reconstructive et Esthetique)
<http://www.plastic-surgery.ch>

This site presents basic information for residents of Switzerland, including site location of surgeons and health insurance. Links to other organizations worldwide are provided for descriptions of surgical procedures. Select English, German, or French to enter this site.

Turkey

Türk Plastik Rekonstrüktif ve Estetik Cerrahi Derneği (Turkish Society of Plastic, Reconstructive and Aesthetic Surgeons)
<http://www.tpcd.org.tr/>

Available in Turkish, with a directory page in English.

United Kingdom (See Great Britain)

Index

9780789010674